21 THINGS
YOU NEED TO KNOW ABOUT
DIABETES

and

NUTRITION

Stephanie A. Dunbar, MPH, RD,
and Cassandra L. Verdi, MPH, RD

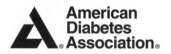

American
Diabetes
Association.

Director, Book Publishing, Abe Ogden; *Managing Editor,* Greg Guthrie; *Acquisitions Editor,* Victor Van Beuren; *Editor,* Lauren Wilson; *Production Manager,* Melissa Sprott; *Composition,* ADA; *Cover Design,* Jody Billert; *Printer,* Versa Press.

Printed in the United States of America
1 3 5 7 9 10 8 6 4 2

The suggestions and information contained in this publication are generally consistent with the Clinical Practice Recommendations and other policies of the American Diabetes Association, but they do not represent the policy or position of the Association or any of its boards or committees. Reasonable steps have been taken to ensure the accuracy of the information presented. However, the American Diabetes Association cannot ensure the safety or efficacy of any product or service described in this publication. Individuals are advised to consult a physician or other appropriate health care professional before undertaking any diet or exercise program or taking any medication referred to in this publication. Professionals must use and apply their own professional judgment, experience, and training and should not rely solely on the information contained in this publication before prescribing any diet, exercise, or medication. The American Diabetes Association—its officers, directors, employees, volunteers, and members—assumes no responsibility or liability for personal or other injury, loss, or damage that may result from the suggestions or information in this publication.

♾ The paper in this publication meets the requirements of the ANSI Standard Z39.48-1992 (permanence of paper).

ADA titles may be purchased for business or promotional use or for special sales. To purchase more than 50 copies of this book at a discount, or for custom editions of this book with your logo, contact the American Diabetes Association at the address below, at booksales@diabetes.org, or by calling 703-299-2046.

American Diabetes Association
1701 North Beauregard Street
Alexandria, Virginia 22311

DOI: 10.2337/9781580405140

Library of Congress Cataloging-in-Publication Data
Dunbar, Stephanie.
  21 things you need to know about diabetes and nutrition / by Stephanie Dunbar and Cassandra Verdi.
     pages cm
  Summary: "By using these healthy tips, this book will help the reader make the connection between healthy eating and managing diabetes"-- Provided by publisher.
  Includes bibliographical references and index.
  ISBN 978-1-58040-514-0 (pbk.)
  1. Diabetes--Diet therapy. 2. Diabetics--Nutrition. 3. Diabetics--Health and hygiene. I. Verdi, Cassandra. II. Title. III. Title: Twenty-one things you need to know about diabetes and nutrition.
  RC662.D86 2013
  616.4'620654--dc23
                    2013010805

DEDICATION

For my parents—thank you for your love and support
and for always being there for me.

—Stephanie

To my mom and dad—for their support, gentle guidance,
and encouragement all of these years.

—Cassie

Table of Contents

Acknowledgments. vii

1 Eating with Diabetes. .1

2 Carbohydrate and Diabetes. 5

3 Best Carbohydrate Choices 11

4 Protein 19

5 Fats 25

6 Meal-Planning Strategies 31

7 Carbohydrate Counting. 37

8 Glycemic Index 43

9 Sweets. 47

10 Artificial Sweeteners .55

11 Beverages 61

12 Alcohol 65

13 Sodium 69

14 Special Occasions 77

15 Breakfast. 81

16 Snacks. 87

17 Eating Out and Quick Meals 93

18 Reading Nutrition Labels. 99

19 Weight Loss. 105

20 Dietary Supplements .111

21 Exercise. 117

    Resources 124

Acknowledgments

There are many people we'd like to thank for their contributions to this book. First, we'd like to recognize Abe Ogden for giving us this unique opportunity to answer the most commonly asked questions about nutrition and diabetes.

A special thanks to Greg Guthrie. We greatly appreciate your patience, kindness, and guidance throughout the writing process. To Victor Van Beuren, for answering many questions along the way and for all of your moral support. To Kelly Rawlings—thank you for sharing your way with words during the writing process. Thanks to Lauren Wilson for doing a wonderful job with copyediting the book—you've been a joy to work with. We'd also like to thank Melissa Sprott for her hard work on the design and layout of this book.

Many thanks to Sue Kirkman, Jane Chiang, and Bob Ratner for the opportunities you have provided and your encouragement and support to expand our work at the Association, including writing this book.

We'd also like to recognize Alison Evert and Sue McLaughlin for their thorough review of this book. We are very grateful for your willingness to share your expert insight into the world of diabetes. A big thank you to Lyn Wheeler for your analysis of our recipes and, more importantly, for being a mentor and lending your time and expertise to advise on many of our projects.

There are many dedicated Association volunteers and colleagues who have contributed to our work at the Association. In doing so you have touched our lives, made our work enjoyable, served as mentors, and become friends. Thanks to all of you.

—*Stephanie and Cassie*

It's impossible not to mention and thank my husband, Jimmy Verdi. You bring so much joy to my life every day, and I am incredibly grateful for your constant encouragement to pursue my dreams.   —*Cassie*

Matthew, thank you for your enthusiasm and your help keeping the book a surprise for a really long time!   —*Mom*

Eating with Diabetes

There are many aspects to managing diabetes. For many people, making food choices is the most challenging. What you eat and how much you eat has a direct effect on your blood glucose level, your risk of developing complications, and many other health factors.

Food is made up of a mix of carbohydrate, protein, and fat. You can think of these as the building blocks for your body. Healthy foods not only provide those building blocks, they provide the extra bonus of vitamins, minerals, and fiber. Choosing healthy foods is the best way to give your body the energy it needs to do daily activities and the things that you love!

Following a healthy, balanced meal plan can help you:

> Lower your A1C (average blood glucose over the past 2–3 months)

> Lower your blood pressure

> Improve your cholesterol levels

> Lose weight or maintain your current weight

> Increase your energy level

> Prevent or delay diabetes complications

What Is a Diabetes Diet?

People often ask which diet is best for managing diabetes. But there is no ideal diet or meal plan that works best for everyone with diabetes. In fact, research has shown that many different ways of eating can work for people with diabetes. The types of meal plans that can be used to manage diabetes include Mediterranean style, low fat, lower carbohydrate, vegetarian, and the DASH (Dietary Approaches to Stop Hypertension) eating pattern.

For people who are overweight, cutting calorie intake is important regardless of the type of meal plan they follow, because it helps with weight loss. Losing a moderate amount of weight can make it easier to control A1C, blood pressure, and cholesterol levels. A moderate amount of weight is about 7% of your body weight. For a person who weighs 200 pounds, for example, that is about 14 pounds.

What Is a Meal Plan?

A meal plan is a guide that tells you how much and what kinds of food to choose at meals and snack times. Some people may refer to a meal plan as an eating plan, food plan, or diet. All of these essentially mean the same thing. Your plan should fit your schedule, culture, and eating habits. The right plan for you should help you keep your blood glucose, blood pressure, cholesterol, and weight on track. For more information on how to create a healthful meal plan, see Chapters 6 (page 31) and 7 (page 37).

Can My Meal Plan Change Over Time?

Yes. Some people with type 2 diabetes are able to control their disease with just diet and physical activity. But over time, many people need to add medications, and sometimes insulin, in order to control their blood glucose. Though people with type 1 diabetes have to take insulin from the start, their needs will change as well. Having to add new medications, change your insulin dose, or adjust your meal plan does not mean that you have failed at managing your diabetes. Most people can expect their health-care provider to make changes to their treatment plan over time.

Tracking your blood glucose level can help you fine-tune your plan. A blood glucose monitor allows you to check your blood glucose level at any point in time. Some providers may have you check your blood glucose at certain times to get an idea of how well your meal plan, exercise routine, and medications are working together. Talk to your health-care provider about whether you should be checking your blood glucose. Those on insulin can especially benefit from this.

Can Healthy Eating Still Taste Good?

Many people assume that eating healthy means giving up all of your favorite treats and restricting yourself to bland meals. This is not true. There are a lot of tasty, flavorful foods and recipes out there that are also good for you. You don't have to eat the same thing every day or give up your favorite foods. It's all about controlling portions and making the best choices *most of the time*.

Who Can Help with Diabetes Meal Planning?

This book will answer some of the most commonly asked questions about nutrition and diabetes. You'll find the information you need to make good food choices and plan diabetes-friendly meals and snacks. We've also included some recipes and practical tips to get you started.

Working one-on-one with a registered dietitian (RD or RDN) is also recommended. Ask your health-care provider if he or she can refer you to an RD who has experience in diabetes or is a certified diabetes educator (CDE). An RD can help you figure out your food needs based on your desired weight, lifestyle, medications, and health goals. Even if you've had diabetes for many years, a visit with an RD can help. Appointments with an RD are covered by many insurance plans.

Diabetes education classes are another option. If you haven't attended a diabetes education class, ask your health-care provider for a referral to a local program. These programs include information on meal planning as well as other components of diabetes care. For now, it's important to learn the basics. Let's get started with what you need to know about including carbohydrate in your meal plan.

Carbohydrate and Diabetes

You've probably heard about carbohydrate if you have diabetes. Many things affect your blood glucose, and one of them is the amount of carbohydrate you eat. Foods with carbohydrate, such as fruits, starchy foods, and dairy products, don't have to be off limits, but knowing how much to eat is important.

How Many Grams of Carbohydrate Can I Eat Each Day?

There is no one amount of carbohydrate that is best for everyone with diabetes. We are all different shapes and sizes, so each person has different needs when it comes to nutrition. The type of diabetes you have, the medications you are on, and many other factors will determine the amount that is best for you.

Blood glucose levels are affected by many factors, including what you eat, when and how much you exercise, available insulin in your body, medicines, hormones, and stress. Of all the foods you eat, those with carbohydrate affect your blood glucose the most. The key to keeping blood glucose levels in your goal range is to balance the food you eat with your physical activity and any pills or insulin you take. If you check your blood glucose, you can use those results to help you fine-tune your meal plan. Finding a way to balance all of these factors is important so you can feel your best, do the things you enjoy, and lower your risk of diabetes complications.

Your health-care team can help you find that balance. Work with them to develop an individualized meal plan that will help you meet your diabetes goals. Your provider can help you set these goals, which might include:

> Losing a certain amount of weight

> Lowering your A1C (average blood glucose over past 2–3 months)

> Lowering your blood pressure

> Improving cholesterol levels

Looking for a Place to Start?

If you haven't set up an individualized plan yet, you can start with a goal of about 45–60 grams of carbohydrate per meal. However, some people may need more and some people may need less. Want more information about carbohydrate counting? Turn to Chapter 7 (page 37).

Work with your health-care team to create the best meal plan for you. Discuss how many grams of carbohydrate to include at each meal and whether or not to include snacks. Over time, you'll learn what works for you and what doesn't.

What Are the Different Types of Carbohydrate?

Did you know there are three main types of carbohydrate in food? They are:

> Starches

> Sugars

> Fibers

You'll also hear terms such as "naturally occurring sugar," "added sugar," "low-calorie sweeteners," "sugar alcohols," "reduced-calorie sweeteners," "processed grains," "enriched grains," "complex carbohydrate," "refined grains," and "whole grains" used to discuss carbohydrate.

No wonder knowing what kind and how much carbohydrate to eat can be confusing!

On the Nutrition Facts label, the term "Total Carbohydrate" includes all three types of carbohydrate. This is the number that you should pay attention to if you are carbohydrate counting.

Starch

You may hear some foods referred to as "starchy." Foods high in starch include:

> Starchy vegetables, such as peas, corn, lima beans, and potatoes.

> Beans, lentils, and peas, such as pinto beans, kidney beans, black-eyed peas, and split peas.

> Grains, such as oats, barley, and rice.

> Bread, pasta, and crackers. (The majority of processed grain products in the U.S. are made from wheat flour but the variety is expanding.) Read more about whole grains in Chapter 3 (page 11).

Sugar

Sugar is another type of carbohydrate. You may also hear sugar referred to as a simple or fast-acting carbohydrate. There are two main types of sugar: naturally occurring sugars, such as those in milk or fruit, and sugars that are added during processing (added sugars). Examples of added sugars include the heavy syrup that fruit is often canned in and the sugar used to make a cookie. On the Nutrition Facts label, the number of sugar grams includes both added and natural sugars.

You may also see table sugar listed by its chemical name: sucrose. The natural sugar in fruit is known as fructose and the sugar in milk is called lactose. You can recognize other sugars on labels because their chemical names also end in "-ose." For example: glucose (also called dextrose), fructose (also called levulose), lactose, and maltose are sugars that you may find listed in the ingredients on a package. For more information on sugar and how it fits into a diabetes meal plan, see Chapter 9 (page 47).

Fiber

Fiber is the indigestible part of plant foods. Fiber-rich foods include fruits, vegetables, whole grains, nuts, and legumes. There is no naturally occurring fiber in animal products, such as milk, eggs, meat, poultry, and fish. When you consume dietary fiber, some types are partially digested, but most of it passes through the intestines and is not digested.

Fiber contributes to digestive health, helps to keep your bowels moving regularly, and makes you feel full and satisfied after eating. Research suggests that there are additional health benefits of a diet high in fiber, such as a reduction in cholesterol levels.

Daily Fiber Recommendations

For good health, adult women should aim for about 25 grams of fiber per day and adult men should aim for about 38 grams per day. Most Americans do not consume nearly enough fiber in their diet, so while it is wise to aim for this goal, any increase in fiber in your diet can be beneficial. Most of us only get about half of the recommended daily amount of fiber.

Good sources of dietary fiber include:

➤ Beans and legumes, such as black beans, kidney beans, pinto beans, chickpeas (garbanzo beans), white beans, and lentils.

➤ Fruits and vegetables, especially those with edible skin (for example, apples and corn) and those with edible seeds (for example, berries).

➤ Whole grains, including:

▷ Whole-wheat pasta, brown rice, whole-grain barley, and quinoa.

▷ Whole-grain cereals (Look for those with 3 grams of dietary fiber or more per serving, including those made from whole wheat and oats. Bran cereals are not whole grain but are very high in fiber and a good choice.)

▷ Whole-grain breads (To be a good source of fiber, one slice of bread should have at least 3 grams of fiber. Another good indication: look for breads where the first ingredient is a whole grain.

For example, whole wheat or oats.) Many grain products now have "double fiber" (extra fiber added).

➤ Nuts and seeds are not high-carbohydrate foods, but are a great source of fiber and healthy fat. Try different kinds such as peanuts, walnuts, almonds, cashews, sunflower seeds, pumpkin seeds, or chia seeds. Just be sure to watch portion sizes because nuts and seeds also contain a lot of calories in a small amount.

In general, an excellent source of fiber contains 5 grams or more per serving. A good source of fiber contains 2.5–4.9 grams per serving.

It is best to get your fiber from food rather than taking a supplement. In addition to the fiber content, fiber-rich foods have a wealth of nutrition and contain many important vitamins and minerals. In fact, they may contain nutrients that haven't even been discovered yet!

If you are not used to eating foods that are high in fiber, gradually increase your fiber intake to prevent stomach irritation. Also, drink more water as you increase your fiber intake, to prevent constipation.

What Is Inulin?

Inulin (not insulin) is a type of fiber that cannot be digested or absorbed. It is added to many food products in the form of chicory root to boost the fiber content. You'll find fiber added to many products, including bread, granola bars, and even yogurt.

Best Carbohydrate Choices

Many people assume that carbohydrate-containing foods are off limits if you have diabetes because they raise blood glucose. However, many carbohydrate-containing foods are also packed with important nutrients that our bodies need to stay healthy. You can still include many carbohydrate foods in your meal plan when you control portions.

What Are the Best Carbohydrate Choices?

When you choose to include carbohydrate-containing foods, make them count! Choose those that are nutrient dense, which means they are rich in fiber, vitamins, and minerals, while also being low in added sugars and unhealthy fats.

Here are the best choices for carbohydrate foods:

➤ Nonstarchy vegetables, such as leafy greens, tomatoes, carrots, cucumbers, and asparagus

➤ Fresh, frozen, or canned fruit without added sugars

➤ Whole grains, such as 100% whole-wheat bread, brown rice, oatmeal, quinoa, and whole-grain barley

- Starchy vegetables, such as sweet potatoes, winter squash, pumpkin, green peas, corn, parsnips, and plantains

- Beans, legumes, and peas

- Low-fat dairy, such as 1% milk, skim milk, and nonfat yogurt

Focus on the foods listed above and limit highly processed carbohydrate foods that provide few nutrients, such as:

- Soda and other sugary drinks

- Refined-grain foods, such as white bread, white rice, many crackers, pastries, and sugary cereals

- Chips, pretzels, and other similar salty snacks

- Sweets and desserts

What Are Nonstarchy Vegetables?

Nonstarchy vegetables are any vegetable with the exception of potatoes, corn, green peas, parsnips, plantains, and most types of winter squash. The best nonstarchy vegetable choices are fresh, frozen, or canned vegetables without added salt, fat, or sugar.

These veggies are packed with important vitamins, minerals, and fiber. They have fewer calories and less carbohydrate than other types of food, so you can actually enjoy them in larger portions. In fact, a good goal to shoot for is to fill at least half of your plate with nonstarchy vegetables at lunch and dinner. Here are just a few ways you could do that:

- Try the recipe for a refreshing Cucumber, Tomato, and Red Onion Salad (page 17).

- Make a salad with spinach, tomatoes, red peppers, radishes, and mushrooms, all drizzled with light dressing.

- Steam broccoli and enjoy it with a squeeze of lemon juice.

- Roast Brussels sprouts that have been lightly tossed in olive oil and seasoned with minced garlic and freshly ground pepper. You could also try roasting other vegetables that you like, such as cauliflower, asparagus, or carrots.

> Steam green beans and top them with a few toasted sliced almonds and trans-fat-free margarine.

> Lightly stir-fry a medley of frozen vegetables.

> Grill sliced eggplant or summer squash that has been lightly brushed with olive oil.

> Lightly sauté your favorite greens with onions and garlic in a little oil. Choose from spinach, kale, or Swiss chard.

> Keep it simple and dip baby carrots and celery sticks in nonfat ranch dressing.

Can I Eat Fruit?

Yes, people with diabetes can still enjoy fruit as part of their daily meal plan. Many people with diabetes are under the impression that they need to avoid fruit because it contains natural sugars. While it does have some carbohydrate from natural sugars, fruit is also high in fiber, vitamins, and minerals, making it a good food choice.

When buying fruit at the store, the best choices are fresh, frozen, or canned fruit without added sugars. Dried fruit and 100% fruit juice are

Budget-Friendly Tips

For a budget-friendly alternative to fresh fruits and vegetables, try frozen and canned varieties. They can be just as nutritious!

For frozen fruits and vegetables—Choose those without added salt, sugar, or sauces.

For canned vegetables—Opt for reduced-sodium varieties when available and be sure to drain and rinse them. This will remove about 40% of the sodium added in the canning process.

For canned fruit—Buy fruit canned in juice if possible. If fruit canned in juice is not available or doesn't fit your budget, buy fruit canned in syrup and drain and rinse it to remove some of the syrup.

also options, but the portion sizes for these options are very small and they are not nearly as filling as fresh, canned, or frozen fruit.

A piece of fruit makes a great snack or side at mealtime. If you are looking for a sweet bite, you could also have fruit to satisfy your craving. It's a much more nutritious dessert choice than cookies or ice cream!

Can I Eat Starchy Foods?

Starchy foods have a place on your plate in small amounts—about 1/4 of your plate. The best starchy food choices are whole grains, beans, and starchy vegetables without added salt, sugar, or fat. Whole grains, beans, and starchy vegetables all contain carbohydrate, but they are great sources of fiber, vitamins, and minerals.

Starchy vegetables are higher in carbohydrate and calories than nonstarchy vegetables, but they can still fit into your meal plan. These include: sweet potatoes, winter squash (with the exception of spaghetti squash), corn, green peas, lima beans, pumpkin, parsnips, and plantains.

Foods such as dried or canned beans, lentils, split peas, black-eyed peas, nonfat refried beans, hummus, and other bean spreads are also good carbohydrate choices. In addition to all the fiber and other nutrients they contain, these foods are also a lean source of protein.

What Counts as a Whole Grain?

The grain group can be split into whole grains and refined grains. Both have about the same amount of calories and grams of carbohydrate in a serving. However, whole grains are a much more nutritious choice than refined grains. Wondering what the difference is?

All grains contain three parts:

> ▸ **The Bran** is the outer hard shell of the grain. It is the part of the grain that provides the most fiber and most of the B vitamins and minerals.

> ▸ **The Endosperm** is the soft part in the center of the grain. It contains the starch.

➤ **The Germ** is technically the seed for a new plant within the grain and is packed with nutrients, including healthy fats and vitamin E.

"Whole grain" means that all three parts of the grain kernel are in the food, so you get all of the nutrients that the grain has to offer. Most refined grains, such as white bread and white rice, have had the most nutritious parts of the kernel (the bran and germ) removed during processing. So you only get the endosperm or the starchy part of the grain, causing you to miss out on a lot of vitamins, minerals, and fiber.

Some common whole grains are:

➤ Bulgur (cracked wheat)

➤ Whole-wheat flour

➤ Whole oats/oatmeal

➤ Whole-grain corn/corn meal/popcorn

➤ Quinoa

➤ Brown rice and wild rice

➤ Whole rye

➤ Whole-grain barley

➤ Whole farro

➤ Buckwheat and buckwheat flour

How do you tell if your bread, pasta, cereal, and crackers are a good source of whole grains? Some of these foods will say that they are "made with whole grain" on the front of the package, when they actually only contain a small amount. For all cereals and grain products, check the ingredient list and make sure one of the grains above is listed first. Many starchy products in the U.S. are wheat based, so most of the time you'll be looking for whole-wheat flour.

Let's Compare

When you choose healthy sources of carbohydrate, you get more nutrients for fewer calories. The portions are often larger and higher in fiber, so you feel full for longer when you choose these foods. Think about it:

Instead of this...	Try this...
1 small blueberry muffin (250 calories, 35 g carbohydrate, 0.7 g fiber)	2/3 cup cooked oatmeal + 2 tablespoons raisins + a sprinkle of cinnamon (170 calories, 35 g carbohydrate, 3.7 g fiber)
15 jellybeans (65 calories, 15 g carbohydrate, 0 g fiber)	1 cup raspberries (65 calories, 15 g carbohydrate, 8 g fiber) OR 1 orange (65 calories, 16 g carbohydrate, 3.6 g fiber)
12-ounce can of soda (150 calories, 40 g carbohydrate, 0 g fiber)	1 peach + 1/2 cup nonfat vanilla Greek yogurt (145 calories, 24 g carbohydrate, 2.3 g fiber)
1.5-ounce bag potato chips (230 calories, 20 g carbohydrate, 1.9 g fiber)	1 cup sugar snap peas + 1/4 cup hummus (165 calories, 17 g carbohydrate, 4 g fiber)

Cucumber, Tomato, and Red Onion Salad

This simple salad makes a great side at dinner and can be a nice change from the traditional salad made with leafy greens.

Serves: 3 / **Serving Size:** 1 cup

1 medium cucumber, peeled and sliced
2 small tomatoes, sliced
1/3 cup sliced red onion
1 tablespoon olive oil
1 tablespoon red wine vinegar
Ground black pepper, to taste

1. In a medium bowl, toss together the cucumber, tomatoes, and red onion.
2. In another small bowl, whisk together the olive oil, red wine vinegar, and ground black pepper.
3. Pour the dressing over the vegetables and toss to coat.
4. Chill the salad in the refrigerator for at least 30 minutes and serve cold.

Nutrition Facts

Calories	65	Potassium	255	mg
Total Fat	4.5 g	Total Carbohydrate	5	g
Saturated Fat	0.7 g	Dietary Fiber	1	g
Trans Fat	0.0 g	Sugars	3	g
Cholesterol	0 mg	Protein	1	g
Sodium	5 mg	Phosphorus	30	mg

Exchanges/Food Choices

1 Vegetable, 1 Fat

Black Bean Quinoa Salad

This whole-grain salad is packed with fiber and is also a good source of protein from the quinoa and beans. Serve it over a bed of leafy greens for a light lunch or as a dinner side with chicken or fish.

Serves: 9 / Serving Size: 1/2 cup

3 cups cooked quinoa
1 (15-ounce) can reduced-sodium black beans, drained and rinsed
2 tablespoons finely diced red onion
1/4 cup chopped cilantro
Juice of 1 lime
1/2 teaspoon fresh ground pepper

1. Combine the quinoa, black beans, red onion, and cilantro in a medium bowl.
2. Pour the lime juice and freshly ground pepper over the other ingredients and toss the salad to mix the ingredients.
3. Serve warm or refrigerate for 30 minutes and serve cold.

TIP: To get 3 cups of cooked quinoa, rinse 1 cup dry quinoa thoroughly with cold water. Combine the rinsed quinoa with 2 cups water in a medium saucepan and bring to a boil. Lower the heat, cover, and simmer for about 12 minutes or until the quinoa has absorbed all the water.

Nutrition Facts

Calories	115		**Potassium**	220 mg
Total Fat	1.5 g		**Total Carbohydrate**	21 g
Saturated Fat	0.2 g		Dietary Fiber	4 g
Trans Fat	0.0 g		Sugars	2 g
Cholesterol	0 mg		**Protein**	5 g
Sodium	55 mg		**Phosphorus**	135 mg

Exchanges/ Food Choices

1 1/2 Starch

Protein

Carbohydrate gets a lot of the attention with diabetes, but it is also important to choose protein foods wisely. The amount of calories and unhealthy saturated fat in protein foods can vary quite a bit. So it's important to choose lean sources of protein and those with healthier fats while also keeping an eye on portion sizes. Including a source of protein can help round out your meal and some people find that it helps them feel full for longer.

Why Is Protein Important?

Protein is found in every cell in your body. It helps us build and repair tissues such as muscles, organs, bones, and skin. You also need protein to make enzymes and hormones, which are essential for many body processes.

What Are the Best Protein Choices?

Many people think that eating meat, poultry, or fish is the only way to get protein in your diet. But there are also many plant-based foods with plenty of protein, such as beans, lentils, and tofu. One benefit of plant-based protein foods is that they are usually lower in unhealthy fats, and may even contain some healthy fats. They also provide fiber, which is not found in animal protein sources. You can find a list of the best animal- and plant-based protein foods below.

> ## Shopping Tip
>
> When shopping for groceries, focus on filling your cart with mostly vegetables (nonstarchy and starchy), fruits, and whole grains. Then pick out some plant-based sources of protein and some fish, poultry, or lean meats (if you eat meat).

Plant-based protein options are a great choice! Choose from:

➤ Beans and legumes (pinto beans, black beans, lentils, black-eyed peas, and garbanzo beans are just a few examples). Try cooking dried beans or using canned beans that have been thoroughly drained and rinsed.

➤ Tofu, tempeh, veggie burgers, soy crumbles, and other soy or gluten-based meat substitutes. Soy milk is a dairy alternative that also provides protein.

➤ Nuts, nut butters, and seeds. These are good sources of protein, and they also provide a good amount of healthy fats. Be sure to watch portion sizes since they are also high in calories.

Good options for animal sources of protein include:

➤ Fish or shellfish.

➤ Low-fat dairy, including 1%, 1/2%, and skim milk, low-fat and nonfat plain or artificially sweetened yogurt. Greek yogurt is even higher in protein than regular yogurt.

➤ Eggs, egg whites, and egg substitutes.

➤ Reduced-fat cheese or cottage cheese.

➤ Poultry, such as chicken, turkey, and Cornish hen *without* the skin.

➤ Lean types of pork, such as pork loin and center loin chops.

➤ Select or Choice grades of beef that have been trimmed of fat, such as chuck, rib, round, rump roast, sirloin, cubed, flank, porterhouse, T-bone steak, tenderloin, or beef jerky.

➤ Veal lean chop or roast.

➤ Lamb chop, leg, or roast.

Limit Processed Meats

Studies have linked processed meats to certain types of cancer, heart disease, and even early death. Processed meats include anything that has been more than cut or ground. Examples are hot dogs, sausage, kielbasa, bacon, and many deli meats, such as bologna, pepperoni, salami, and pastrami. The takeaway? When choosing animal sources of protein, go with fresh instead of processed sources.

A lot of us have been raised to plan our meals around the meat on our plate with small sides of vegetables. But over the years, more and more research has supported the value of eating more plant-based foods and less red and processed meats in the diet to control weight and reduce disease risk.

The Diabetes Plate Method described in Chapter 6 (page 31) can serve as a guide to help you control your meat portions. It's an easy way to see if you are getting enough vegetables too.

Portion Control Tip

A serving of fish, poultry, or meat is 3–4 ounces, which is about the size of a woman's palm or a deck of cards.

Plant-Based Protein

Plant-based or vegetarian eating plans are becoming increasingly popular. It's easy to make a delicious, well-rounded meal with vegetarian protein. Plant-based protein foods, such as tofu and beans, are naturally lower in unhealthy saturated and trans fats than animal-based protein.

Don't be afraid to give meatless meals a chance! Choose a vegetarian entrée when you go out to eat. Or, start by cooking at least one meatless meal each week. Some ideas are stir-fry with tofu, veggie burgers, or 3-bean veggie chili topped with a dollop of plain Greek yogurt.

Tips for Selecting and Preparing Protein Foods

▶ For chicken or turkey, the white breast meat is leaner than the dark meat of the bird. If you're looking for a less expensive cut, opt for chicken or turkey legs or thighs. Always remove the skin from all cuts to reduce the amount of unhealthy fat and calories.

▶ Cut away all visible fat on meats and choose the cut with the least amount of visible fat/marbling.

▶ When selecting ground beef or ground turkey, choose those marked as 90% lean or more. For the leanest option, try 99% lean ground turkey breast.

▶ If you are on a budget you can still buy the less expensive, higher-fat ground beef. Just drain the fat after cooking and rinse the cooked beef with hot water.

▶ Buying lean meats, poultry, or fish in bulk can be a money saver. They freeze well, so you can use what you need and freeze the extras for another day. Most uncooked meat or poultry can be stored in the freezer for 3 months or more.

Fish and Omega-3 Fatty Acids

You've probably heard about fish and heart-healthy omega-3 fatty acids. Omega-3s are a type of healthy fat that helps lower cholesterol levels. Fish are a good source of omega-3s, especially those that are considered "fatty fish." Healthy fatty fish that are high in omega-3 fatty acids include: salmon, herring, trout, sardines, mackerel, and albacore tuna. Try to include fish, particularly fatty fish, in your meal plan at least two times per week.

Get your omega-3s from fish and natural food sources rather than supplements, which have not been shown to reduce your risk of heart disease. For more information, see Chapter 20 (page 111) on supplement use. Want to learn more about healthy fats? Turn to Chapter 5 (page 25).

Shopping Tip

For convenience, try buying frozen fish, which may also be a less expensive option than buying fresh fish.

Simple Oven-Roasted Salmon

Here is a quick and simple fish recipe that's high in protein and healthy fats. Serve it with a side of brown rice and steamed green beans.

Serves: 4 / **Serving Size:** 1/4 recipe

Cooking spray
4 fresh salmon fillets (about 4 ounces each or 1 pound total)
1 tablespoon olive oil
1 teaspoon dried dill
1/4 teaspoon freshly ground pepper
2 teaspoons lemon juice

1. Preheat the oven to 425°F and coat a glass baking dish with cooking spray.
2. Lay the salmon fillets in the baking dish and brush the top of each fillet with olive oil.
3. Sprinkle dill and ground pepper evenly over each fillet and roast in the oven for 10–12 minutes, or until the fish is opaque and flakes when touched with a fork.
4. After removing the fish from the oven, pour lemon juice evenly over each fillet and serve immediately.

Nutrition Facts

Calories	230	Potassium	360	mg
Total Fat	13.0 g	Total Carbohydrate	0	g
Saturated Fat	2.2 g	Dietary Fiber	0	g
Trans Fat	0.0 g	Sugars	0	g
Cholesterol	80 mg	Protein	25	g
Sodium	60 mg	Phosphorus	255	mg

Exchanges/Food Choices

4 Lean Protein, 1 1/2 Fat

Fats

For a long time, we thought that a low-fat diet was the answer to reducing heart disease risk and losing weight. Many people still think that it is best to limit how much fat we eat. It is true that fat is high in calories, but more recent research shows that certain types of fat, when eaten in moderate amounts, may actually promote health. Because people with diabetes are at increased risk for cardiovascular disease, it's a good idea to limit the unhealthy fats you eat and replace some of them with healthier fats. At the same time, you should keep your portions of healthy fats small to avoid excess calories, especially if you are trying to lose weight.

Healthy Fats Explained

What makes a type of fat healthy versus unhealthy? And which foods are the best sources of healthy fat? Two types of healthy fat you may have heard of are polyunsaturated fats and monounsaturated fats. These unsaturated fats may help improve cholesterol levels and reduce your risk for heart disease. Omega-3 fatty acids are a type of polyunsaturated fat that has been found to promote heart health. Find out which foods are sources of these healthy fats in the chart below:

Monounsaturated Fat	Polyunsaturated Fat	Omega-3 Fatty Acids
Olives and olive oil Canola oil and peanut oil Nut butters and nuts (like almonds, cashews, pecans, peanuts) Avocado Sesame seeds	Walnuts, pumpkin seeds, and sunflower seeds Other oils such as saf-flower, soybean, corn, cottonseed, and sunflower Trans-fat-free soft margarine, mayonnaise, and salad dressings	Fatty fish, such as salmon, mackerel, halibut, herring, albacore tuna, sardines, anchovies, and rainbow trout Plant-based sources such as English walnuts and walnut oil, flaxseeds and flaxseed oil, soybean products and soybean oil, and chia seeds.

Which Fats Are Considered "Unhealthy"?

Some fats are detrimental to our health and raise our cholesterol levels. Try to limit the amount of the following fats in your diet:

➤ Trans fat

➤ Saturated fat

Limit Trans Fats

Trans fat is made by a process called hydrogenation, which turns liquid oil into solid fat. Trans fat is the worst type of fat. It raises total cholesterol and LDL cholesterol, increasing your risk for heart disease and stroke. It's best to limit the trans fat in your meal plan as much as possible. The U.S. Food and Drug Administration (FDA) is currently considering eliminating all artificial trans fat from the food supply, so hopefully, trans fats will no longer be found in foods in the near future.

You'll find trans fat in stick margarines, shortening, some processed snacks and baked goods, some brands of peanut butter, and some fast foods and fried foods. Use the Nutrition Facts label and ingredient list to check if these foods contain trans fat.

It is important to know that food companies can claim 0 grams of trans fat on the Nutrition Facts label as long as a food has less than 0.5

grams per serving. Take extra caution and check the ingredient list for partially hydrogenated oil or hydrogenated oil, which are other names for trans fat. If you see either listed, that means the food has some trans fat in it even if the label says it has 0 grams of trans fat. Be cautious about eating foods with these ingredients as even small amounts can add up quickly.

Reduce Saturated Fat in Your Meal Plan

Saturated fat is another type of unhealthy fat. The American Diabetes Association recommends limiting saturated fat to no more than 10% of your total calories. When cutting back on foods high in saturated fat, you can replace them with foods that are higher in healthy fats.

Use the Nutrition Facts label to see how much saturated fat is in the foods you buy. Cut back on how often you have these foods and keep portion sizes small when you do choose them. Foods that are high in saturated fat include:

➤ High-fat dairy, such as full-fat cheese, cream, ice cream, whole milk, 2% milk, and sour cream

➤ High-fat meats, such as regular ground beef, bologna, hot dogs, sausage, bacon, and spareribs

➤ Lard, butter, or fatback

What's the Deal with Chocolate?

You may have heard that chocolate is a heart-healthy food. However, it is also a source of saturated fat. Claims such as this can be confusing when making food choices. Many of the studies that have looked at chocolate and heart health have used a type of chocolate much higher in cocoa and flavonoids than what you'll find in a typical milk chocolate bar. (Flavonoids are thought to protect against heart disease and cancer.)

The takeaway? When you want a chocolate treat, opt for dark chocolate, which has a higher cocoa and flavonoid content than milk chocolate. Also, remember to keep portions small. All chocolate is dense in calories and it's easy to eat a lot of calories in a small serving. Savor one piece to enjoy the flavor and curb your sweet tooth. Remember that a square of dark chocolate on occasion can be an enjoyable treat, but don't depend on it to contribute significantly to heart health.

- Cream-based sauces

- Gravy made with meat drippings

- Palm oil and palm kernel oil

- Coconut and coconut oil

- Poultry (chicken and turkey) skin

Simple Tips to Include More Healthy Fats and Fewer Unhealthy Fats

Here are some practical ways you can fit in more healthy fats and reduce the saturated and trans fat in your meal plan. (Don't forget that healthy fats are still high in calories and need to be eaten in moderate amounts.)

- Cook with plant-based oils, such as olive, peanut, or canola oil instead of butter, margarine, shortening, or lard.

- Instead of processed snacks (e.g. chips, pretzels, and cookies), choose snacks such as nuts, natural peanut butter spread on fruit, or fresh veggies with salad dressing or guacamole.

- Currently drinking 2% or whole milk? Try making the switch to 1% milk or even skim. You can also try fortified soy milk or almond milk.

- Instead of using cream, try a lower-fat milk in your coffee.

- Trim any visible fat from meats and remove skin from turkey and chicken before cooking.

- Instead of meat for dinner, switch it out for some heart-healthy salmon or tuna. You could also choose a vegetarian option, such as veggie burgers or grilled Portobello mushrooms.

- Choose reduced-fat cheese rather than full-fat cheese. If you don't like reduced-fat varieties, halve the amount of full-fat cheese that you add to your food.

- Choose low-fat or nonfat yogurt topped with sliced fruit for dessert instead of chocolate, candy, or baked goods.

> Instead of flavoring vegetables with creamy sauces or butter, try using a small drizzle of olive oil, freshly ground pepper, and garlic to add extra flavor. Trans-fat-free margarines are also an option.

> Trade the bacon on your omelet or burger for some fresh avocado slices.

Key Takeaways

> Cut back on foods high in unhealthy fats, and replace them with sources of healthy fats.

> Watch portion sizes, even with healthy fats, since all fats are dense in calories.

Homemade Balsamic Vinaigrette

Make your own salad dressing at home and you'll eliminate a lot of the sodium and other additives that are found in store-bought dressing.

Serves: 3 / **Serving Size**: 2 tablespoons

1/4 cup balsamic vinegar
2 tablespoons olive oil
1/2 teaspoon Dijon mustard
1/4 teaspoon ground pepper

1. In a small bowl, whisk all dressing ingredients until combined.

Nutrition Facts

Calories	100	**Potassium**	25	mg
Total Fat	9.0 g	**Total Carbohydrate**	4	g
Saturated Fat	1.2 g	Dietary Fiber	0	g
Trans Fat	0.0 g	Sugars	3	g
Cholesterol	0 mg	**Protein**	0	g
Sodium	25 mg	**Phosphorus**	0	mg

Exchanges/Food Choices

2 Fat

4-Ingredient Guacamole

Have guacamole as a snack with whole-wheat crackers, baby carrots, or cucumber rounds. You can also use it as a topping on tacos, burgers, and sandwiches. It's high in heart-healthy monounsaturated fats from the avocado!

Serves: 4 / **Serving Size:** 1/4 cup

1 medium avocado
Juice of 1/2 lime
2 tablespoons canned, chopped green chilies
2 tablespoons finely diced red onion

1. Peel avocado and remove the pit.
2. In a medium bowl, partially mash avocado so that some small chunks remain.
3. Stir in lime juice, green chilies, and red onion.

> **TIP:** If you like a kick, add crushed red pepper to taste. If you want to mix it up, you could also add 1/4 cup chopped fresh tomatoes for very few additional calories and carbohydrate.

Nutrition Facts

Calories	65	**Potassium**	210	mg
Total Fat	6.0 g	**Total Carbohydrate**	5	g
Saturated Fat	0.8 g	Dietary Fiber	3	g
Trans Fat	0.0 g	Sugars	1	g
Cholesterol	0 mg	**Protein**	1	g
Sodium	20 mg	**Phosphorus**	25	mg

Exchanges/ Food Choices

1 Vegetable, 1 Fat

Meal-Planning Strategies

One of the first questions a person usually asks when they are diagnosed with diabetes is: "What can I eat?" Your health-care provider may have suggested that you change how you eat but you weren't sure how to do that. The easiest way to plan meals and control portions is to use the Diabetes Plate Method. You don't need any special tools for this portion control method and you don't need to count carbs or calories. It's simple, effective, and you can use it anywhere.

Get started building a healthier plate by following these seven simple steps:

1. Draw an imaginary line across the middle of a 9-inch plate. Then on one half, draw another line down the middle. You will have three sections on your plate.

2. Fill the largest section with nonstarchy vegetables, such as salad, green beans, broccoli, cauliflower, carrots, and tomatoes.

3. In one of the small sections, put starchy foods, such as bread, rice, pasta, corn, beans, and potatoes.

4. The other small section is for protein foods, such as chicken, fish, lean meat, tofu, and eggs.

5. Add a piece of fruit, a cup of milk or yogurt, or both as your meal plan allows.

6. Choose healthy fats in small amounts. For cooking, use oils. For salads, some healthy additions are nuts, seeds, avocado, and vinaigrettes.

7. To complete your meal, add a glass of water, unsweetened tea, or coffee.

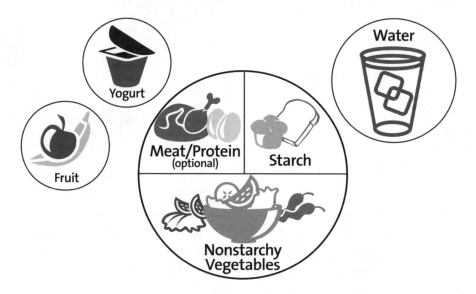

You can still enjoy your favorite foods by changing how much you eat. Your plate may include more nonstarchy vegetables and less protein and starchy foods, but you'll still be able to fit in your favorite foods in the correct portion sizes.

The Diabetes Plate Method helps you keep the amount of carbohydrate you eat about the same at each meal, which may help you manage blood glucose levels. This method also makes it easier to determine if your portion of starch is too big or if you are eating enough vegetables. To learn more about the best food choices for each section of your plate, see Chapters 3, 4, and 5.

Add Variety

Feel like you are filling your plate with the same foods every day? Try some of the foods in the lists below to add variety to your meals.

Nonstarchy Vegetables—1/2 of Your Plate

- Asparagus
- Beets
- Bok choy
- Broccoli
- Brussels sprouts
- Cabbage
- Cauliflower
- Carrots
- Cucumber
- Eggplant
- Green beans
- Mushrooms
- Onions
- Okra
- Pea pods and snap peas
- Peppers
- Pico de gallo
- Spaghetti squash
- Spinach, kale, Swiss chard, other leafy greens
- Tomatoes and tomato sauce
- Turnip
- Zucchini or summer squash

Protein Foods—1/4 of Your Plate

- Fish, such as salmon, tuna, tilapia, and cod
- Other seafood, such as shrimp, scallops, oysters, crab, and mussels
- Tofu, tempeh, or veggie burgers or nuggets
- Chicken or turkey (skin removed)
- Cheese or cottage cheese
- Ground turkey breast or 90% lean ground beef
- Eggs, egg whites, or egg substitute
- Pork tenderloin, center loin chop, ham, or Canadian bacon
- Beef sirloin, top round, bottom round, or eye of round, trimmed of visible fat

Starchy Foods—1/4 of Your Plate

- Brown or wild rice, quinoa, bulgur, couscous
- Whole-grain barley or farro
- Whole-wheat roll, pita, or pasta
- Corn tortilla or naan
- Potatoes, sweet potatoes, or parsnips
- Cooked beans or peas, such as chickpeas, pinto beans, black beans, and black-eyed peas
- Nonfat refried beans, hummus, or dal
- Corn, green peas, lima beans
- Winter squash (pumpkin, acorn, butternut)

(continued)

(continued from p 33)
Fruit—on the Side

> ➤ Apple, apricot, banana, grapefruit, grapes, kiwi, mango, papaya, peach, pear, pineapple, plum, or orange

> ➤ Berries, such as blackberries, blueberries, raspberries, and strawberries

> ➤ Melon, such as cantaloupe, honeydew, and watermelon

Dairy—on the Side

> ➤ Milk: skim, 1/2%, or 1%
> ➤ Unflavored, fortified soy, rice, or almond milk

> ➤ Nonfat plain yogurt (regular or Greek yogurt)
> ➤ Nonfat light flavored yogurt (regular or Greek yogurt)

Water or Low-Calorie Drink

> ➤ Unsweetened teas
> ➤ Coffee
> ➤ Club soda

> ➤ Other low-calorie drinks and drink mixes, such as light lemonade and diet soda

How Can I Control My Portions?

Controlling portions can be difficult. The portions of food and beverages available in packages and served in restaurants have increased significantly over time, making it tough to judge how much we should be eating. Using the Diabetes Plate Method to control your portions is a great place to start. Here are other ways to keep your portions in perspective.

Does the Size of Your Dishes Matter?

Not only have the portions served at restaurants increased, but so has the size of plates and glasses in our homes. It is easy to serve and eat large portions without realizing it if you use large plates, bowls, and glasses. By using smaller dishes, it seems like you are eating more.

Take a minute to find out how much food and drink your dishes hold. How many inches is your plate across the middle? The plate used for the Diabetes Plate Method should be 9 inches in diameter. Most new plates in the store are at least 11 inches across. If you have large plates, you may want to find some smaller ones. Try eating off a smaller plate, or avoid filling your plate to the edges, to see if it helps you reduce portion sizes.

Take a look at the bowls in your kitchen. Do they hold 1 cup of cereal or is it closer to 2 cups? Measure out what 1 cup of cereal or soup looks like in the bowls you have at home, and keep that in mind when using them. Wide, shallow soup bowls usually hold less but will give the impression that you are eating just as much.

The shape of a glass can trick your eye so it looks like you are drinking more or less depending on the shape. A tall, thin glass looks like it holds more than a short fat glass. So when having milk, juice, or anything that is not calorie free, use a tall thin glass to help control your portion. Small juice glasses usually hold more than 1 cup. Many larger glasses hold 3 cups. If you fill a large glass with juice, it is about 360 calories and 90 grams of carbohydrate! For more information on beverages, see Chapter 11 (page 61).

Use Simple Ways to Estimate Portions

When food labels, measuring cups, or small dishes are not available, use these guidelines to estimate portion sizes:

- ➤ 3 ounces of fish, chicken, or meat = 1 deck of cards or woman's palm

- ➤ 1/2 cup = half a baseball

- ➤ 1 cup = closed fist or baseball

- ➤ 1 tablespoon = thumb

- ➤ 1 teaspoon = thumb tip

Portions 20 Years Ago vs. Now*

Keeping an eye on your portions is key for diabetes management. Our idea of what portion sizes look like has changed significantly over the past 20 years—especially when eating out. Even if you are selecting healthy foods, if you eat too much, you are sabotaging your efforts for managing your weight (if that is one of your goals) and improving your glycemic control.

	20 Years Ago	Today
Bagel	3 inches in diameter	6 inches in diameter
	140 calories	350 calories
Muffin	1.5 ounces	4 ounces
	210 calories	500 calories
Popcorn	5 cups	11 cups
	210 calories	630 calories
Cookie	1.5 inches in diameter	3.5 inches in diameter
	55 calories	275 calories
Spaghetti and Meatballs	1 cup spaghetti with sauce and 3 small meatballs	2 cups of pasta with sauce and 3 large meatballs
	500 calories	1,025 calories
French Fries	2.4 ounces	6.9 ounces
	210 Calories	610 Calories
Soda	6.5 ounces	20 ounces
	85 Calories	250 Calories
Turkey Sandwich	320 calories	820 calories

*Adapted from NHLBI Portion Distortion Quizzes

Carbohydrate Counting

Carbohydrate counting, or "carb counting," is a meal planning technique for managing your blood glucose levels. Carbohydrate counting helps you keep track of how much carbohydrate you are eating. With carbohydrate counting, you set an amount or range of carbohydrate to eat for a meal. The right balance of physical activity and medicine (if you take it) can help you keep your blood glucose levels in your target range.

Finding the right amount of carbohydrate depends on factors such as how active you are and what, if any, medicines you take. The foods you choose to eat are up to you as long as you eat the amount of carbohydrate that is right for you. For more information on how much carbohydrate to eat, see Chapter 3 (page 11).

Why Worry About Carbohydrate?

The key to keeping blood glucose levels in your target range is to balance the food you eat with your physical activity and any pills or insulin you take. The carbohydrate in food makes blood glucose levels go up. If you eat more carbohydrate than usual, it is more likely that your blood glucose levels will be higher than usual after a meal. Likewise, if you eat less than usual, you would expect your blood glucose levels to be lower in comparison. Finding the balance for yourself is important so you can feel your best, do the things you enjoy, and lower your risk of diabetes complications.

Planning Meals

There are two popular ways to plan meals when you have diabetes.

> Carbohydrate counting
> Diabetes Plate Method

Something to consider when you decide which method is best for you is the type of medication you take (if any). If you take multiple injections of insulin every day, you can have more flexibility in when and how much you eat if you use carbohydrate counting.

If you are "diet controlled" and use diet and exercise to manage diabetes, using the Diabetes Plate Method to keep your carbohydrate intake consistent may be very useful. You can find more information about using the Diabetes Plate Method in Chapter 6 (page 31).

Where Should I Start?

1. The first step is to learn which foods contain carbohydrate. Carbohydrate-containing foods include:

> Starchy foods, such as bread, cereal, rice, and crackers

> Fruit and juice

> Milk and yogurt

> Beans, like pinto beans, and other plant-based proteins, like veggie burgers

> Starchy vegetables, such as potatoes and corn

> Sweets and snack foods, such as sodas, cake, cookies, candy, and chips

Nonstarchy vegetables have a little bit of carbohydrate, but in general are very low in carbohydrate.

2. Next, learn how much carbohydrate is in different foods. Once you know which foods contain carbohydrate, you can start to use labels and portion sizes to count the carbohydrate in your meal. Reading Nutrition Facts labels is a great way to know how much carbohydrate is in a food. To learn more about reading Nutrition Facts labels, see Chapter 18 (page 99). When a food does not have a label, you have to estimate the amount of carbohydrate in it. When you get started with carbohydrate counting, measuring your foods will help you estimate how much carbohydrate you are eating.

For example, there are about **15 grams of carbohydrate** in:

> ➤ 1 small piece of fresh fruit (4 ounces)
> ➤ 1/2 cup of canned or frozen fruit
> ➤ 2 tablespoons of dried fruit
> ➤ 1/2 cup fruit juice
> ➤ 1 slice of bread (1 ounce) or 1 (6-inch) tortilla
> ➤ 1/2 cup of oatmeal
> ➤ 1/3 cup of pasta or rice
> ➤ 4–6 crackers
> ➤ 1/2 English muffin or hamburger bun
> ➤ 1/2 cup of black beans or starchy vegetables
> ➤ 1/4 of a large baked potato (3 ounces)
> ➤ 2/3 cup of nonfat yogurt (plain or sweetened with sugar substitutes)
> ➤ 2 small cookies
> ➤ 2-inch square brownie or cake without frosting
> ➤ 1/2 cup ice cream or sherbet
> ➤ 1 tablespoon syrup, jam, jelly, sugar, or honey
> ➤ 2 tablespoons light syrup
> ➤ 6 chicken nuggets
> ➤ 1/2 cup of casserole
> ➤ 1 cup of soup
> ➤ 1/4 serving of a medium order of french fries

Counting Nonstarchy Vegetables

Nonstarchy vegetables have about 5 grams of carbohydrate in 1 cup of raw or 1/2 cup of cooked vegetables. Therefore, they are not usually counted unless you have three portions or more at one time.

3. Decide how \much carbohydrate to have at each meal.

Finding the right amount of carbohydrate for you can take a little bit of trial and error. As described in Chapter 2 (page 5), some people start with about 45 grams of carbohydrate for a meal and then adjust. Some people will eat more and some will eat less. The amount you eat might not be the same for all meals of the day. (For example, you might eat less at breakfast than at other meals.) You should talk to your health-care provider about the amount of carbohydrate that is right for you.

4. Now you're ready to plan a meal. Here's an example.

If you want to plan a meal with about 45 grams of carbohydrate, think about what foods you plan to eat. If you plan to have chicken, rice, spinach with salad dressing, and canned peaches, here are the steps:

➤ Identify the foods with carbohydrate. Rice and peaches contain carbohydrate.

➤ You know that 1/3 cup of rice has about 15 grams of carbohydrate.

➤ You know that 1/2 cup of peaches has about 15 grams of carbohydrate.

➤ You decide to eat 2/3 cup of rice and 1/2 cup of peaches.

   ▷ 2/3 cup of rice = 30 grams of carbohydrate

   ▷ 1/2 cup canned peaches = 15 grams of carbohydrate

   ▷ This totals to about 45 grams of carbohydrate.

➤ You can then balance your carbohydrate foods with protein (chicken) and healthy fats (salad dressing drizzled on the spinach).

Balance with Protein and Healthy Fats

With carbohydrate counting, it is easy to forget about the protein and fat in your meals. To balance your meals, include a source of lean protein and healthy fats at each meal. For more information on making the best food choices, see Chapter 4 on protein (page 19) and Chapter 5 on fats (page 25).

Using Nutrition Facts Labels

Carbohydrate counting is easier when Nutrition Facts labels are available. You can look at how much carbohydrate is in the foods you want to eat and decide how much to eat based on your plan. The two most important things to look for on a label when carbohydrate counting are the serving size and the amount of total carbohydrate.

> ➤ Look at the Serving Size. All the information on the label is about this amount of food. If you will be eating a larger portion, then you will need to double or triple the information on the label, as appropriate.

> ➤ Look at the grams of Total Carbohydrate.

>> ▷ "Total Carbohydrate" on the label includes sugar, starch, and fiber.

>> ▷ Know the amount of carbohydrate you can eat, and figure out the portion size to match.

See Chapter 18 (page 99) for more information on reading Nutrition Facts labels.

If I Use Insulin, Do I Have To Eat the Same Amount of Carbohydrate at Each Meal?

If you take insulin, you may be able to have more flexibility in how much carbohydrate you eat at each meal. This is called matching your insulin to your carbohydrate intake.

People who use insulin are trying to mimic the way their body would normally release insulin. In people without diabetes, the pancreas releases a small amount of insulin all the time. This is called basal insulin. When people without diabetes eat, the pancreas releases enough insulin to keep blood glucose normal as the food is digested and absorbed. This spurt of insulin is called a bolus.

There are two types of insulin that people with diabetes use to replace the insulin that their pancreas doesn't make.

> Long-acting insulin: It mimics the basal insulin release.

> Fast-acting insulin: It mimics a bolus of insulin release.

Some people with diabetes adjust their amount of fast-acting insulin based on how much carbohydrate they eat. If you are taking the same amount of fast-acting insulin every time you have a meal, talk to your health-care team about whether you can have some flexibility.

A great brochure that teaches how to have a more flexible carbohydrate counting schedule, *Match Your Insulin to Your Carbs,* can be purchased at www.shopdiabetes.org.

Glycemic Index

The glycemic index (GI) measures how a carbohydrate-containing food raises blood glucose. To determine the GI, foods are ranked based on how they compare to a reference food—either glucose or white bread. A food with a high GI raises blood glucose more than a food with a medium or low GI. People typically eat several foods at a meal, so the after-meal glucose level is affected by the combination of foods and by the person's available insulin.

Meal planning with the GI involves choosing foods that have a low or medium GI. If eating a food with a high GI, you can combine it with low-GI foods to help balance the meal. Examples of carbohydrate-containing foods with a low GI include dried beans and legumes (such as kidney beans and lentils), all nonstarchy vegetables, some starchy vegetables (such as sweet potatoes), most fruit, and many whole-grain breads and cereals (such as barley, whole-wheat bread, and all-bran cereal). Meats and fats don't have a GI because they do not contain carbohydrate.

Following is a list of foods categorized by their GI.

Low-GI Foods

➤ 100% stone-ground whole-wheat or pumpernickel bread

➤ Oatmeal (rolled or steel-cut), oat bran, muesli

➤ Pasta, converted rice, barley, bulgur

➤ Sweet potato, corn, yam, lima/butter beans, peas, legumes, and lentils

➤ Most fruits, nonstarchy vegetables, and carrots

Medium-GI Foods

➤ Whole-wheat, rye, and pita bread

➤ Quick oats

➤ Brown, wild, or basmati rice and couscous

High-GI Foods

➤ White bread or bagel

➤ Corn flakes, puffed rice, bran flakes, instant oatmeal

➤ Short-grain white rice, rice pasta, macaroni and cheese from mix

➤ Russet potato, pumpkin

➤ Pretzels, rice cakes, popcorn, saltine crackers

➤ Melons and pineapple

What Is the Glycemic Load?

The glycemic load is a measure that takes into account the amount of carbohydrate and the glycemic index of a food.

What Affects the GI of a Food?

As a general rule, the more cooked or processed a food, the higher the GI; however, this is not always true. Fat and fiber also tend to lower the

GI of a food. Below are a few specific examples of other factors that can affect the GI of a food:

> Individual response: not everyone has the same blood glucose response to a food.

> Ripeness and storage time: the more ripe a fruit or vegetable is, the higher the GI.

> Processing: juice has a higher GI than whole fruit, mashed potatoes have a higher GI than whole baked potatoes, and regular whole-wheat bread has a higher GI than stone-ground whole-wheat bread.

> Cooking method: how long a food is cooked can affect the GI (al dente pasta has a lower GI than soft-cooked pasta).

> Variety: converted long-grain white rice has a lower GI than brown rice, but short-grain white rice has a higher GI than brown rice.

Other things to consider if using the GI:

> The GI can be difficult to use because we do not label our foods with the GI in the U.S.

> The GI value represents the type of carbohydrate in a food but says nothing about the amount of carbohydrate typically eaten. Portion sizes are still important for managing blood glucose and for losing or maintaining weight.

> The GI of a food is different when the food is eaten alone than when it is combined with other foods. When eating a high-GI food, you can combine it with low-GI foods to balance out the effect on blood glucose levels.

> Many nutritious foods have a higher GI than foods with little nutritional value. For example, oatmeal has a higher GI than a candy bar. But that does not make the candy bar a healthy choice. You should still focus on healthful food choices if using the GI.

Is the GI a Better Tool Than Carbohydrate Counting?

There is no one diet or meal plan that works for everyone with diabetes. The important thing is to follow a meal plan that is tailored to your personal preferences and lifestyle and helps you achieve goals for blood glucose, cholesterol and triglyceride levels, blood pressure, and weight management.

Research shows that both the amount and the type of carbohydrate in foods affect blood glucose levels. Studies also show that the total amount of carbohydrate in food, in general, is a stronger predictor of blood glucose response than the GI. Based on the research, for most people with diabetes, the first tool for managing blood glucose is some type of carbohydrate counting. For more information on carbohydrate counting, see Chapter 7 (page 37).

But because the type of carbohydrate affects blood glucose, using the GI may be helpful in "fine-tuning" blood glucose management. In other words, combined with carbohydrate counting, the GI may provide an additional benefit for achieving blood glucose goals for individuals who can and want to put extra effort into monitoring their food choices.

Some individuals may find it helpful to create their own personal GI list of foods. By checking your blood glucose before and after eating, you can identify how certain foods affect your blood glucose. For example, if you eat 30 grams of carbohydrate from pasta, you can see how that compares to eating 30 grams of carbohydrate from rice. If you check your blood glucose, share these results with your health-care team.

Sweets

9

Can I Eat Sugar and Desserts?

People with diabetes can still enjoy small amounts of sugar and dessert. In the past, people with diabetes were told to completely avoid sugar. People thought that eating sugar would raise blood glucose levels very high. Now experts agree that you can substitute small amounts of sugar-containing foods for other carbohydrate-containing foods in your meals. Having dessert is no longer considered "cheating"—it's a choice.

The total amount of carbohydrate you eat affects blood glucose levels more than the type of carbohydrate. That doesn't mean you can eat all the sugar or dessert you may want. (No one should do that, whether they have diabetes or not!) Most sweets contain a large amount of carbohydrate and calories in a very small serving, so you need to be sure to keep portions small.

Sweets and desserts don't provide the important vitamins and minerals found in more healthful carbohydrate foods, and they are often higher in fat and calories. So, you'll want to save them for special occasions instead of making them part of your daily meal plan.

Sugar Has Many Names

There are many types of sweeteners besides table sugar that have calories and carbohydrate. You should treat all of these sugars the same way in your meal plan. Examples are:

- Table sugar (also called white sugar or sucrose)
- Raw sugar
- Cane sugar
- Sugar cane syrup
- Beet sugar
- Honey
- Brown sugar
- Molasses
- Fructose
- Maple syrup
- Cane sugar
- Agave nectar
- Confectioners' sugar
- Powdered sugar
- Turbinado
- High fructose corn syrup (also called corn sugar)
- Rice syrup or brown rice syrup
- Coconut palm sugar

How Much Carbohydrate Is Found in Common Desserts?

A small portion of dessert can have a lot of carbohydrate. Here is a list comparing the carbohydrate content of common desserts to healthier carbohydrate-containing foods:

- About 15 grams of carbohydrate
  - ▷ 1/2 cup ice cream = 1 1/4 cup of strawberries
- About 30 grams of carbohydrate
  - ▷ 1 small piece of frosted cake (2-inch square) = 1/2 an English muffin with 1 tablespoon of peanut butter and 1 plum
- About 45 grams of carbohydrate
  - ▷ Fruit pie with crust (1/6 of 8-inch pie) = 1 cup of blueberries and 3/4 cup of cereal and 1/2 cup of milk
- About 60 grams of carbohydrate
  - ▷ Large cookie (6 inches wide) = 6 cups of popcorn, 1 cup of light yogurt, and an orange

Many sugars are labeled as "natural" or as having a low glycemic index. This can be very confusing. Keep in mind while you are reading labels, that all of the above types of sugar contain about the same amount of carbohydrate per teaspoon. Each teaspoon has about 4 grams of carbohydrate whether you are using white sugar, beet sugar, or agave nectar. All of these sweeteners need to be counted in your meal plan, regardless of marketing claims that a product has a low glycemic index.

How Do I Include Dessert in My Meal Plan?

The key to keeping your blood glucose levels on target is to substitute small portions of sweets and sweeteners for other carbohydrate-containing foods in your meals and snacks. The idea is to eat about the same amount of carbohydrate as you normally would.

Carbohydrate-containing foods include (but are not limited to):

- bread
- cereal
- yogurt
- tortillas
- fruit
- potatoes
- rice
- juice
- corn
- crackers
- milk
- peas

To include sweets in your meal, you can cut back on other carbohydrate-containing foods at the same meal.

For example, if you'd like to have cookies with your lunch, you need to substitute them for another carbohydrate-containing food. If your lunch is a turkey sandwich made with two slices of bread, here are the steps you would take to make the substitution:

1. Your first step is to identify the carbohydrate-containing foods in your meal. Bread and cookies both contain carbohydrate.

2. Use the Nutrition Facts label to determine how many grams of carbohydrate are in a slice of bread and a serving of cookies.

3. Swap or replace a slice of bread for an equal amount of carbohydrate in the cookies.

4. It's an even trade. Your total amount of carbohydrate remains the same for the meal.

Skip the Everyday Temptations

Everyone has their favorite treats that they've enjoyed for many years. But we are surrounded by an abundance of dessert foods, such as packaged cookies, candy bars, prepackaged cupcakes, and pies. Our suggestion? Keep these packaged desserts from the grocery store out of your pantry so you aren't tempted to snack on them. Save your dessert for something you really enjoy and look forward to on special occasions. Another idea is to buy one slice of pie or cake from your local bakery or store instead of bringing home the whole pie or cake.

Better-for-You Fruit and Dairy Desserts

Think beyond cakes and cookies. Pick a dessert with a touch of decadence that satisfies your sweet craving and helps you sneak in some extra fruit or dairy servings. Some great better-for-you desserts are:

➤ A baked apple

➤ Low-fat fruit cobbler

➤ Low-fat pudding

➤ A yogurt and berry parfait

➤ A couple of pieces of fruit dipped in dark chocolate

➤ Grilled fruit

Key Takeaways

You can have dessert. Try to save it for special occasions and only indulge in your favorites. When you *do* decide to include a treat, keep portions small and swap this treat for other carbohydrate foods in your meal plan.

Quick Cinnamon Baked Apple

There is nothing easier than turning an ordinary piece of fruit into a delicious dessert.

Serves: 2 / **Serving Size:** 1/2 apple

1 medium apple (macintosh or other cooking apple)
2 teaspoons whipped butter
1 teaspoon brown sugar
1/2 teaspoon ground cinnamon

1. Peel and core the apple and cut it in half.
2. Put 1 teaspoon of whipped butter in the center of each apple half.
3. Sprinkle each apple half with 1/2 teaspoon of brown sugar.
4. Sprinkle the apples with cinnamon.
5. Bake in the oven at 375°F for 15–20 minutes until apple is soft.
6. Serve warm.

Nutrition Facts

Calories	60		**Potassium**	65	mg
Total Fat	2.0 g		**Total Carbohydrate**	11	g
Saturated Fat	1.2 g		Dietary Fiber	1	g
Trans Fat	0.0 g		Sugars	9	g
Cholesterol	5	mg	**Protein**	0	g
Sodium	15	mg	**Phosphorus**	10	mg

Exchanges/Food Choices

1/2 Fruit, 1/2 Fat

Chocolate-Dipped Walnuts and Apricots

Satisfy your chocolate craving with dark chocolate, walnuts, and dried apricots.

Time: 10 minutes
Serves: 5 / **Serving Size:** 2 walnut halves + 2 apricots

1 ounce dark chocolate
10 walnut halves
10 dried apricots

1. Melt the dark chocolate in the microwave for 30 seconds, stir, and microwave for an additional 15–30 seconds until melted.
2. Dip one end of each walnut half and one end of each dried apricot in melted chocolate.
3. Lay dipped pieces on wax paper to harden. To speed up the hardening process, put the dipped fruit and nuts in the refrigerator.
4. Once chocolate has cooled and hardened, remove from wax paper and store in an airtight container.

Nutrition Facts

Calories	90	**Potassium**	210	mg
Total Fat	4.5 g	**Total Carbohydrate**	12	g
Saturated Fat	1.6 g	Dietary Fiber	2	g
Trans Fat	0.0 g	Sugars	10	g
Cholesterol	0 mg	**Protein**	1	g
Sodium	0 mg	**Phosphorus**	40	mg

Exchanges/Food Choices

1 Carbohydrate, 1 Fat

Yogurt and Berry Parfait

Beautiful presentation can turn ordinary foods into a sweet treat.

Serves: 2 / Serving Size: 1 parfait

1 teaspoon honey
1 cup nonfat plain Greek yogurt
2 cups berries

1. Mix the honey with the yogurt.
2. In a parfait dish, wine glass, or goblet, layer 1/3 cup berries, 1/4 cup yogurt, 1/3 cup berries, and 1/4 cup yogurt. Finish with an additional 1/3 cup berries on top. Repeat this process in a second glass or parfait dish.

Nutrition Facts

Calories	140		**Potassium**	335	mg
Total Fat	0.5	g	**Total Carbohydrate**	22	g
Saturated Fat	0.0	g	Dietary Fiber	4	g
Trans Fat	0.0	g	Sugars	17	g
Cholesterol	0	mg	**Protein**	13	g
Sodium	45	mg	**Phosphorus**	180	mg

Exchanges/Food Choices

1 Fruit, 1 Fat-Free Milk

Artificial Sweeteners

Can Someone with Diabetes Use Artificial Sweeteners?

People with diabetes can use artificial sweeteners if they choose to do so. Sometimes artificial sweeteners are also called low-calorie sweeteners, sugar substitutes, or non-nutritive sweeteners. They can be used instead of sugar to sweeten foods and drinks for fewer calories and less carbohydrate.

All of the artificial sweeteners that are available have been reviewed by the U.S. Food and Drug Administration (FDA) and determined to be safe for everyone, including people with diabetes. It is a personal choice whether or not you use them. Some people find them useful for adding a touch of sweetness for less carbohydrate than sugar. Others prefer to have a smaller portion of dessert without low-calorie sweeteners. The choice is yours.

What Are the Different Types of Artificial Sweeteners?

There are several types of artifical sweeteners. Common examples include:

- Acesulfame potassium (also called acesulfame K)
- Advantame
- Aspartame
- Neotame

- Stevia (also called rebaudioside A, reb-A, or rebiana)
- Saccharin
- Sucralose
- Monk fruit

These sweeteners are used by food companies to sweeten diet drinks, baked goods, frozen desserts, candy, light yogurt, and chewing gum. You can also buy them to use as tabletop sweeteners. You have probably seen some of the name brands such as Splenda, Sweet 'N Low, TruVia, or Equal, but many stores also carry generic brands of these sweeteners, which tend to cost less. You can add them to coffee or tea or sprinkle them on top of oatmeal. The sweetening power of most artificial sweeteners is at least 100 times more intense than regular sugar, so only a small amount is needed when you use these sugar substitutes. Some are also available in "granular" versions that can be used in cooking and baking.

Do Artificial Sweeteners Contain Carbohydrate?

Yes, they can. The sweetener itself is calorie free; however, to make the product look similar to sugar, additional ingredients are added to the pure sweeteners for texture and volume. These ingredients (some common ones are dextrose and maltodextrin) will also add a small amount of calories and carbohydrate to the product.

When reading food labels, remember that foods are considered "no-calorie" if they have 5 calories or fewer per serving. Low-calorie sweeteners claim zero calories and carbohydrate on the Nutrition Facts label; however, there is a small amount of calories and carbohydrate from the added ingredients. When you use a large amount of these products, it can add up. As with all foods, it is important not to go overboard.

The following list shows how many calories and carbohydrate are in one packet of common low-calorie sweeteners. For comparison, one packet of sugar has 11 calories and 3 grams of carbohydrate.

Sweetener	Calories	Carbohydrate (grams)
1 packet Splenda (sucralose)	4	<1
1 packet Sugar Twin (saccharin)	3	<1
1 packet Equal (aspartame)	4	<1
1 packet SweetLeaf (stevia)	0	0

In addition to individual packets, some artificial sweeteners are available in large quantities for baking purposes. There are several versions of artificial sweeteners made for baking, including brown sugar versions, plain granular versions, or premixed blends of sugar and artificial sweetener. Pay attention to the type you are buying, as the carbohydrate content and use in sweetening foods and beverages can be significantly different. Always read labels carefully so you know how much carbohydrate is in the product on the shelves.

Cooking with Artificial Sweeteners

If you decide to use sugar substitutes when baking or cooking, there are a few important things to know:

> Baked products may be lighter in color because real sugar has a caramelizing/browning effect and artificial sweeteners do not.

> Volume may be lower in cakes, muffins, and quick breads because artificial sweeteners do not have the same bulking ability as sugar.

> Texture may be altered in some baked products, especially cookies.

> Taste may be slightly different if you are sensitive to the sweetener's aftertaste.

> Cooking time of your baked goods may be slightly different when using artificial sweeteners.

> Sugar naturally holds in moisture and increases keeping quality, so baked products with the sugar removed will not keep as long.

> There may be specific instructions for using artificial sweeteners for baking or cooking. Read the package carefully for information on the best way to substitute the artificial sweetener for sugar in your recipes. The company's website can also be a helpful resource for baking tips.

Can I Eat as Much Sugar-Free Food as I Want?

No, many foods labeled "sugar-free," "reduced sugar," or "no sugar added" are not calorie or carbohydrate free. They may not even be lower in carbohydrate than the original version. You should not eat as much as you want because they will still raise blood glucose just like any other type of carbohydrate food.

Always check the Nutrition Facts label, even for foods that carry these claims. Low-calorie sweeteners are often used in foods in place of sugar; however, many of these foods still contain a significant amount of calories, total carbohydrate, and fat. As an example, a slice of fruit pie labeled "no sugar added" still has a large amount of carbohydrate, fat, and calories in one serving. "No sugar added" means there is no *extra* sugar added. But the other ingredients still count! Some products may contain less carbohydrate and you need to read labels carefully to identify products that may be useful to you. Remember that all types of carbohydrate will affect blood glucose levels, and sugar is only one type of carbohydrate.

Sugar on Nutrition Facts Labels

Sugar is listed under "Total Carbohydrate" on the Nutrition Facts label. Keep in mind that this amount includes both added sugars and naturally occurring sugars, such as the natural sugar in raisins or milk.

It is helpful to check the total carbohydrate amount because *it includes both sugar and starch*. If you only look at the sugar content, you are not accounting for the starch in a food. This means you could be underestimating how much a food will raise your blood glucose. For more on reading Nutrition Facts labels, see Chapter 18 (page 99).

What Are Sugar Alcohols?

Sugar alcohols are a type of reduced-calorie sweetener. Despite the name "sugar alcohols," they do not contain alcohol. You can find them in ice creams, cookies, puddings, candies, and chewing gums that are labeled as "sugar-free" or "no sugar added." Sugar alcohols provide fewer calories than sugar and have less of an effect on blood glucose than other sources of carbohydrate.

The grams of sugar listed on the label do not include any sugar alcohols that may be in the product. It is voluntary for food manufacturers to list sugar alcohols on the label. However, the amount of total carbohydrate on the Nutrition Facts label does include sugar alcohols. If a food doesn't list sugar alcohols separately on the label, you can look for individual sugar alcohols in the ingredient list. Look for ingredients that end in "-ol," such as maltitol or sorbitol. Most sugar alcohols still contain some carbohydrate and calories.

Examples of sugar alcohol are:

- Erythritol
- Glycerol (also known as glycerin or glycerine)
- Hydrogenated starch hydrolysates
- Isomalt
- Lactitol
- Maltitol
- Mannitol
- Sorbitol
- Xylitol

Please note: Sugar alcohols can have a laxative effect or cause other gastric symptoms in some people, especially in children. If you find that you experience these symptoms, you may need to limit the amount of sugar alcohols in your diet.

Key Takeaways

Foods with artificial sweeteners can have fewer calories than foods made with sugar. However, many of the food products containing these types of sweeteners still have a significant amount of carbohydrate, calories, and fat. Never consider them a "free food" without checking the label. By comparing the Nutrition Facts label of the sugar-free version of a food to that of the regular version, you'll see if you're really getting fewer calories and less carbohydrate and fat with the sugar-free product.

Beverages

Making smart drink choices is just as important as making smart food choices. What you drink can have a big impact on your weight, your blood glucose, and your overall health. What's more, research has shown that liquid calories do not give us the same "full" feeling that we get from solid food. So stick to zero-calorie and very-low-calorie drinks, such as:

> Water (tap, carbonated, mineral, or with a squeeze of lemon or lime juice)

> Teas (iced or hot; unsweetened or sweetened with a low-calorie sugar substitute)

> Coffee (black or sweetened with a low-calorie sugar substitute)

> Club soda

> Diet sodas

> Other sugar-free drinks like light lemonade and low-calorie drink mixes

Drinks to Avoid

Sugary drinks include regular soda, fruit punch, juice drinks, energy drinks, sports drinks, sweet tea, and regular lemonade, which are all high in calories and carbohydrate. These are drinks you'll want to avoid. Some sugary drinks, such as lattes and specialty coffee drinks, have added sugar and unhealthy fats in them.

It doesn't matter if they are sweetened with sugar, high-fructose corn syrup, agave nectar, or another type of sugar—these drinks can cause blood glucose to rise. They can also provide several hundred calories in just one serving! Those calories will add up and cause weight gain over time if you drink these every day. Use this list to compare the calories and carbohydrate content of a few sugary drinks to zero-calorie drinks:

➤ 1 standard size can of cola (12 fluid ounces or 1 1/2 cups) = about 140 calories + 40 grams of carbohydrate

➤ 1 cup (8 fluid ounces) of fruit punch and many fruit drinks = 100 calories (or more) + 30 grams of carbohydrate

➤ 1 cup (8 fluid ounces) of water or diet drink = 0 calories + 0 grams of carbohydrate

Milk and Juice

Low-fat milk and 100% juice can also be healthy drink choices in the right portions. Portion size is very important, especially for juice, because the portion size for one serving is very small. It is only about 1/3–1/2 cup. These drinks have calories and carbohydrate, but they also provide important vitamins and minerals. When you choose these drinks, be sure to check Nutrition Facts labels for the portion size and amount of carbohydrate in a serving so you can count them in your meal plan.

For milk, choose 1%, 1/2%, or skim. Avoid flavored milks with added sugar. If you are lactose intolerant or if you don't like milk, fortified unflavored soy, rice, or almond milk are all great substitutes to try.

If you choose to buy juice, choose 100% juice with no added sugar. If you want some juice, check the Nutrition Facts label to determine the portion size that will fit with your meal plan. If you like to have juice in the morning but don't want all of the carbohydrate from it, another option is low-sodium vegetable juice, which has just 50 calories and 10 grams of carbohydrate in 1 cup. Keep in mind that eating fruits and vegetables is a better choice than juice. It is very easy to consume 3 servings (and 45 grams of carbohydrate) from juice. Whole fruits and vegetables are more filling, provide fiber, and make you less likely to eat more than one portion.

Functional Beverages

There are many different types of energy drinks and vitamin waters available. These drinks are often called "functional beverages," which means they contain added ingredients such as extra vitamins, minerals, and herbs. Often, these ingredients are advertised to have certain health benefits. The labels on these beverages may have claims such as "promotes heart health," "promotes immunity," or "increases energy."

It is best to approach these drinks with caution. If you choose to drink them, always check the Nutrition Facts labels. Does your drink of choice contain calories and carbohydrate? Is it sweetened with added sugars? If so, it may not be the best choice. Energy drinks are controversial right now. Many of these have significant amounts of caffeine and other stimulants that may be harmful.

Beware of the claims you see on labels—particularly for drinks that are marketed as being good for diabetes. These may be false or taken out of context. These products are usually expensive and are not essential to managing diabetes. Even if you use functional beverages, it is still important to follow a healthy meal plan, be physically active, and take any medications that have been prescribed for you.

Are Caffeinated Beverages Safe?

You might be wondering if you can still have caffeine and whether or not it will affect your blood glucose level. While a few small studies have looked at caffeine/coffee consumption and the effect on blood glucose, there is not enough research to discourage people with diabetes from drinking coffee or other caffeinated drinks in moderation.

According to the American Medical Association, three 8-ounce cups of coffee (about 250 milligrams of caffeine total) per day or five servings of caffeinated tea is considered a moderate amount of caffeine, and is not likely to have a negative impact on health if you have an otherwise healthy lifestyle. Coffee and tea (without added milk, cream, or sweeteners) are very-low-calorie drinks with less than 5 calories per cup and no carbohydrate.

Caffeine Caution

If you experience side effects such as insomnia or arrhythmias after drinking regular coffee or tea, it is probably a good idea to switch to decaf coffee and tea. Herbal teas that are labeled "caffeine free" are also a great option.

Be cautious of specialty coffee drinks, such as lattes and mochas. Unlike regular, unsweetened coffee, they can provide a significant amount of fat, carbohydrate, and calories in your meal plan. If you decide to treat yourself to one of these drinks, use these tips when you order:

➤ Ask for your drink to be made with nonfat or skim milk. Many coffee shops automatically use 2% or whole milk unless you ask.

➤ Forgo the whipped cream, caramel, or other sweet toppings. These drinks are flavorful enough on their own!

➤ Check the nutrition information in the store or online before ordering to see which drinks will work with your meal plan.

➤ Ask for the smallest size. Is there an 8-ounce option rather than the typical 12-ounce drink?

➤ Ask if sugar-free syrup is available for the type of drink you choose. This can help you cut down even more on calories and carbohydrate.

Wondering what to do when it comes to alcoholic drinks? Find more information in Chapter 12 (page 65).

Alcohol

Can I Drink Alcohol If I Have Diabetes?

Most people with diabetes can include a moderate amount of alcohol in their meal plan. In fact, some research has shown that there are health benefits to having one drink per day. Still, there are some people who should use caution when drinking. If you have been told by your health-care professional to avoid alcohol, you should follow his or her instructions.

What Does "Drinking in Moderation" Mean?

Drinking in moderation means having no more than one drink per day for women and no more than two drinks per day for men. All of the following have about the same amount of alcohol and are considered one drink or serving.

> ➤ 1 1/2 ounces of liquor or spirits
> ➤ 5 ounces of wine
> ➤ 12 ounces of beer

Are There Benefits to Alcohol?

Moderate amounts of alcohol have been shown to reduce the risk of heart disease. Some studies have also shown that a regular, moderate intake of alcohol may lower A1C. Both are good news for people with diabetes. But before you decide that a half bottle of wine or a six-pack of beer is back on the menu, consider that studies also show that drinking more than one to two drinks per day can increase your risk of heart disease and some cancers. Like most everything, a little alcohol can be good, but too much can be a problem. The key is to be safe and stick to the rules of moderation.

How Much Does Your Glass Hold?

Do a reality check on your glassware at home and at your favorite restaurant spots. Most wine glasses hold two servings (10 ounces) of wine or more if they are full. Measure what a serving looks like in your glasses at home and make a mental note of it. A standard bottle or can of beer is 12 ounces, but a pint of beer at your favorite pub is 16 ounces—and that is just the regular size!

Who Should Avoid Alcohol?

There are some people who should not drink:

> People with alcohol abuse problems

> People with poor glycemic control or severe episodes of hypoglycemia, at least until blood glucose management has improved

> People with certain complications, such as nephropathy. Symptoms can worsen when drinking alcohol. Talk to your health-care provider if you are not sure if alcohol is safe for you.

> Children and adolescents

> Pregnant women

Most people who take insulin or insulin secretagogues (pills that help your body release more insulin) can include a moderate amount of alcohol in their meal plan with a few extra precautions. Alcohol is processed differently than food and can cause low blood glucose levels up to 24 hours after drinking. Eating food when you drink is important to prevent hypoglycemia if you use insulin or insulin secretagogues. Checking your blood glucose while you're drinking and the day after consuming alcohol is recommended to see how alcohol affects you.

Tips to Stay Safe While Drinking

➤ Always wear identification, such as medic alert jewelry, that says you have diabetes, especially if you use diabetes medicines such as insulin or insulin secretagogues. Symptoms of low blood glucose or hypoglycemia (such as confusion, lack of coordination, and light-headedness) are similar to signs of being tipsy or intoxicated.

➤ Always drink in moderation and make sure someone you are with knows the signs and symptoms of low blood glucose and can help you treat it.

➤ Check with your health-care team about whether it is safe for you to drink alcohol, especially if you are taking medicine for diabetes or other medical conditions.

➤ Check your blood glucose levels to see how alcohol affects you on the night of the event and the next day.

➤ Always eat food if you drink an alcoholic beverage. Because of the calories in alcoholic beverages, many people try to cut back on their food intake. This is a mistake and can increase your risk of severe hypoglycemia for up to 24 hours after drinking—particularly if you take insulin or a pill that lowers blood glucose levels.

➤ Stick to no more than two drinks per day for men and no more than one drink per day for women. (A drink is 12 ounces of beer, 1 1/2 ounces of distilled spirits, or 5 ounces of wine.)

➤ Mixed drinks, sweet wine, beer, and liqueurs (such as Irish crème, Schnapps, or Amaretto) can contain carbohydrate in addition to the alcohol. When possible, use sugar-free mixers, such as diet tonic water, light cranberry juice, or diet sodas, if having a mixed drink. Some other light options to consider are wine spritzers and light beer.

➤ If you drink on a regular basis, talk with your health-care team about how to include alcohol in your meal plan.

Sodium

Why Does the Amount of Sodium in My Diet Matter?

In many people, sodium intake is linked to increased blood pressure and an increased risk of having a stroke. In other words, the more sodium you eat and drink, the more likely it is that your blood pressure will be high.

Sodium has been a hot topic lately, and recommendations from the government as well as several national health organizations are encouraging people to consume less sodium. Sodium has been used to preserve foods for centuries. It was a critical component added to keep foods safe to eat before refrigeration. But in recent years, the amount of sodium found in most packaged and processed foods has continued to increase.

Where Does the Sodium in Our Diet Come From?

Most people think that the salt they add to their cooking or to food at the table is the biggest source of sodium in their diet. This is actually not true! Most of the sodium that people eat in the U.S. comes from processed and restaurant foods. On average, only about 11% of the sodium Americans eat comes from the salt shaker. The biggest single source of sodium is actually bread products, which don't even taste salty! Of course, many other types of processed foods are high in sodium as well. Here are some examples:

- Canned soups, vegetables, and meats
- Pickled foods
- Salad dressings and marinades
- Frozen dinners and pizza
- Processed meats, such as turkey, ham, and roast beef deli meats
- Cheeses
- Sauces and soy sauce
- Chips and pretzels

On the other hand, fresh foods, such as fresh lean meats, fruits, vegetables, plain brown rice, and plain oats, are very low in sodium. To reduce the amount of sodium you eat, fresh food choices are always best.

What Is the Difference Between Salt and Sodium?

Salt and sodium are not the same thing, but you will hear them used interchangeably. Salt is found in nature and its chemical name is sodium chloride. So, technically, salt is only about half sodium. One teaspoon of salt has 2,300 mg of sodium. That is enough sodium for one whole day all by itself without considering the sodium content of processed foods.

How Much Sodium Should I Eat in a Day?

The American Diabetes Association recommends that everyone with diabetes try to consume less than 2,300 mg of sodium per day. If you have high blood pressure, your health-care provider may want you to have even less.

How Can I Cut Back on Sodium?

Fortunately, there are many easy ways to cut back on sodium. Eating less processed food and filling up on fresh food instead is the key. When you think about food and wonder if something is processed, think about whether your ancestors a century ago would recognize what you are about to eat. If not, it is probably processed.

The good news is that many foods that are naturally low in sodium require no cooking and are your best options for snacking. Try fresh fruit, unsalted nuts, and easy-to-pack veggies, such as cherry tomatoes, baby carrots, and snap peas, for snacks instead of highly processed foods, such as chips and crackers.

There are some processed foods, such as canned vegetables, that can be easily switched for those that have less added sodium. If your budget doesn't allow for the lower-sodium variety, thoroughly drain and rinse canned vegetables and beans to reduce the sodium by about 40%. For other canned or boxed foods, reading labels can help you find foods with less sodium. Restaurant and fast foods are often very high in sodium. For tips on making healthier restaurant choices, see Chapter 17 (page 93).

Reducing the amount of salt you add to foods is another way to cut back on sodium, and it doesn't have to be difficult. You can gradually cut back on salt in your cooking to allow your taste buds to adjust. It can take several weeks to get used to the way things taste with less salt. As you decrease the salt in your food, try using spices and herbs to bring different flavors into your food. Try spices and herbs such as chili powder, garlic, cilantro, parsley, fresh ground pepper, basil, curry powder, ginger, rosemary, or thyme. Other ways to flavor food include using vinegar, garlic, or fresh lemon or lime juice.

Budget-Friendly Tips

> Drain and rinse canned vegetables.
> Choose frozen vegetables without sauces.
> Buy fresh fruits and vegetables when they're on sale. Often they are cheaper and on sale when in season.
> Buy whole grains, such as plain rice, barley, farro, and quinoa. Buying the plain grains instead of mixes saves you money and drastically cuts the sodium. These grains are naturally low in sodium and can be flavored easily with spices, herbs, lemon juice, and nuts.
> Cook fresh turkey and freeze the cooked leftovers. You can thaw the turkey to use in sandwiches instead of deli meats.

Citrus Walnut Rice

You can make your own nutritious "rice mix" at home for less sodium. Here are a few variations to try.

Serves: 2 / Serving Size: 1/2 cup

1 cup cooked brown rice or brown rice medley
2 teaspoons dried parsley
2 tablespoons finely chopped walnuts
1 tablespoon lemon juice

1. Cook the rice according to package instructions, omitting any salt.
2. Add parsley, walnuts, and lemon juice.
3. Stir and serve hot.

Nutrition Facts

Calories	160		**Potassium**	95	mg
Total Fat	6.0	g	**Total Carbohydrate**	24	g
Saturated Fat	0.6	g	Dietary Fiber	2	g
Trans Fat	0.0	g	Sugars	1	g
Cholesterol	0	mg	**Protein**	4	g
Sodium	10	mg	**Phosphorus**	110	mg

Exchanges/Food Choices

1 1/2 Starch, 1 Fat

Quick Cumin Rice

Serves: 2 / Serving Size: 1/2 cup

1 cup cooked brown and wild rice medley
1/4 teaspoon cumin
1/2 teaspoon freshly ground black pepper
2 tablespoons finely chopped onion

1. Cook the rice according to package instructions, omitting any salt.
2. Add cumin, pepper, and onion.
3. Stir and serve hot.

Nutrition Facts

Calories	110	**Potassium**	200 mg
Total Fat	1.5 g	**Total Carbohydrate**	22 g
Saturated Fat	0.1 g	Dietary Fiber	2 g
Trans Fat	0.0 g	Sugars	1 g
Cholesterol	0 mg	**Protein**	3 g
Sodium	345 mg	**Phosphorus**	80 mg

Exchanges/Food Choices

1 1/2 Starch

Fresh Salsa

Salsa is often recommended as a lower-calorie and lower-carbohydrate dip for chips and tacos. But store-bought salsa is usually quite high in sodium, with 2 tablespoons of salsa having over 200 mg of sodium. But you're in luck—homemade salsa is quick and simple to make!

Serves: 8 / Serving Size: 1/4 cup

1 large tomato, chopped
3/4 cup diced onion
1 clove garlic, crushed
1 jalapeño pepper, diced
3/4 cup chopped fresh cilantro, large stems removed
3 tablespoons lime juice (juice of 1 lime)

1. Combine chopped vegetables and cilantro and mix together. Add lime juice to mixture and stir.
2. Store in the refrigerator for 2 hours to allow flavors to mix.
3. Use as a dip for tortilla or pita chips, mix it with rice, or use it as a topping for grilled fish or chicken.

Nutrition Facts

Calories	15	Potassium	110	mg
Total Fat	0.0 g	**Total Carbohydrate**	3	g
Saturated Fat	0.0 g	Dietary Fiber	1	g
Trans Fat	0.0 g	Sugars	2	g
Cholesterol	0 mg	**Protein**	1	g
Sodium	0 mg	**Phosphorus**	15	mg

Exchanges/Food Choices

Free food

Variations for making fresh salsa are unlimited. See page 75 for more ideas.

Fruity Fresh Salsa

If you like fruity salsa, add 1 cup chopped or canned diced mango to the Fresh Salsa recipe (page 74).

Serves: 12 / Serving Size: 1/4 cup

Nutrition Facts

Calories	18	Potassium	95	mg
Total Fat	0.0 g	Total Carbohydrate	4	g
Saturated Fat	0.0 g	Dietary Fiber	1	g
Trans Fat	0.0 g	Sugars	3	g
Cholesterol	0 mg	Protein	0	g
Sodium	0 mg	Phosphorus	10	mg

Exchanges/Food Choices

Free food

Fresh Corn Salsa

Cook 1/2 cup of frozen corn, drain, and add to Fresh Salsa recipe (page 74) for a flavorful side dish.

Serves: 10 / Serving Size: 1/4 cup

Nutrition Facts

Calories	18	Potassium	100	mg
Total Fat	0.0 g	Total Carbohydrate	4	g
Saturated Fat	0.0 g	Dietary Fiber	1	g
Trans Fat	0.0 g	Sugars	1	g
Cholesterol	0 mg	Protein	1	g
Sodium	0 mg	Phosphorus	15	mg

Exchanges/Food Choices

Free food

Special Occasions

There are many situations—such as changes in your daily schedule, demands at work, holiday events, parties, and travel delays—that can disrupt your meal plan. And on super busy days, sometimes eating is the last thing on your mind. Planning in advance can help you prepare for special events and ensure that your kitchen is stocked with quick meals and snacks.

Planning for Parties and Holiday Meals

Parties and holiday celebrations can be a time of worry for people with diabetes. Not only are many events focused on food, but also the timing of the meal may not match up to your usual schedule.

If you take insulin injections on a fixed schedule or medication that lowers blood glucose, delayed meals can lead to low blood glucose. If your meal will be later than usual—perhaps you're planning to eat at a party or are going to a restaurant—you may need to eat a snack at your normal mealtime to prevent a low blood glucose reaction. Then enjoy your usual amount of food, for a meal, during the party. Check with your health-care team about whether there are any special precautions you should consider.

Expect Travel Delays and Always Carry Snacks

Airport travel (and even travel by train or car) can be stressful. Delays are inevitable and having snacks on hand will help keep you from skipping meals and keep temptation for less healthy choices at bay. Some snacks that are easy to slip into your carry-on and will make it through airport security without any problems include nuts, an apple or grapes, whole-grain crackers, granola bars, or a peanut butter sandwich.

If your travel plans don't include airports, you have even more snack options, including canned vegetable juice, yogurt, sandwiches, and cheese that you can stock in a small cooler. Save money on drinks by bringing a reusable, empty water container. Bottled water is usually marked up in the airport and will cost you about $3. Instead of purchasing water, fill up your water bottle at a drinking fountain. For a bit of flavor, stash a few single-serving, sugar-free drink mixes in your bag.

Many airport eateries, both fast-food and sit-down restaurants, are offering healthier choices these days. If your travels are long, you will likely need a bite to eat during the trip, so do a bit of research online to see what is available at your layover destination. Keep these tips for eating out in mind while traveling:

➤ Order the smallest sandwich without cheese and sauce.

➤ Get all sauces and dressings on the side.

➤ Split something if entrées are large.

➤ Order a lunch portion if available.

➤ Avoid fried foods and sides.

➤ Ask for a salad or vegetables instead of fries.

For more information on eating out, see Chapter 17 (page 93).

Too Busy for Lunch?

Don't think you have enough time to eat lunch? Try some of these tips:

1. Keep nonperishable foods at work or even in your car to have when there is no time to pack a lunch. Prepacking to-go foods in single-serving portions can help you control your portions and save money. Eat them later while you are on the go. Here are some foods you can grab quickly as you leave for the day:

   > Whole-wheat crackers

   > Nuts and seeds

   > Flavored popcorn cakes or soy chips

   > Dried fruit

   > Beef jerky

   > Canned tuna

   > Peanut butter

   > Small cans of 100% vegetable juice

   > Single-serving containers of fruit, such as canned peaches, mandarin oranges, fruit cocktail, or applesauce

   > Meal replacement bars or shakes

2. If you have a refrigerator at work, you have more options. Keep these foods on hand or even pack them on the weekend for the week ahead:

   > Reduced-fat cheese

   > Hard-boiled eggs

   > Hummus

   > Baby carrots, snap peas, or cherry tomatoes

   > Whole fruits, such as oranges, apples, or pears

   > Yogurt or cottage cheese

   > Leftovers

3. If you have time to pack lunch the night before, here are some more options for a healthy, well-balanced meal:

   > Put a healthy spin on the traditional sandwich: use two pieces of

thin sandwich bread, 2 ounces of reduced-sodium lean turkey, hummus, spinach, bell pepper, and mustard. Add some carrot sticks and light ranch dressing on the side.

▶ Mix together some cooked quinoa, white beans, chopped bell pepper, carrots, and broccoli to make a grain salad. Toss with a teaspoon of olive oil, a teaspoon of lemon juice, salt, and pepper. Add a nectarine or some grapes on the side and a small handful of dry-roasted almonds, if desired.

▶ Make a tuna salad with canned tuna, light mayo, diced celery, lemon juice, and freshly ground pepper. Serve 1/2 cup of tuna salad over greens with a sliced apple and 2 tablespoons of peanut butter on the side.

▶ Try a quick yogurt parfait. Mix 1 cup of nonfat plain Greek yogurt, 1/2 cup diced pineapple or peaches, and a small handful of pecans.

▶ Pack 1 cup of leftover chili or vegetable soup. Top it with some fresh tomatoes and a spoonful of nonfat plain Greek yogurt instead of sour cream.

▶ Fill a whole-wheat tortilla wrap with a couple slices of rotisserie chicken, 1–2 tablespoons hummus, sundried tomatoes, a sprinkle of feta cheese, and greens. Add a piece of fruit if it fits with your plan.

▶ Try a hard-boiled egg with a piece of fruit, a string cheese, and 5 whole-wheat crackers. You could also add some carrots, celery sticks, and 1–2 tablespoons of peanut butter.

▶ Toss together a salad with romaine lettuce or spinach and any other nonstarchy vegetables that you like. Top it with some low-fat cottage cheese, 1/4 cup of chopped nuts, and a tablespoon of light dressing.

▶ Wrap a few slices of leftover rotisserie chicken and leftover salad in a whole-wheat tortilla.

Key Takeaways

1. Plan ahead for special occasions or travel.
2. Stock your kitchen for quick meals and snacks.
3. Keep nutritious, non-perishable foods at work or in your car.

Breakfast

Why Eat Breakfast?

It can be helpful for people with diabetes to follow a regular eating pattern. When you spread your carbohydrate intake throughout the day and avoid skipping meals, it's easier to keep your blood glucose under control.

Having a healthy breakfast can set the tone for your day. Some studies have also linked regular breakfast eating to having a healthier body weight, increased concentration, and increased energy levels.

What If I'm Not Hungry in the Morning?

You don't have to eat breakfast immediately after waking. However, it is important to eat something when you start to feel hungry. If you wait too long to eat between meals, it can lead to overeating later on. Make sure you eat something when you get hungry and stick to the meal plan you've worked out with your health-care team.

How Much Carbohydrate Should I Have at Breakfast?

The amount of carbohydrate you eat at each meal will depend on your individual meal plan. For some people, it may be best to have less carbohydrate at breakfast (say, 30 grams or less). Others may be able to have closer to 60 grams of carbohydrate in the morning without compromising their blood glucose levels. If you check your blood glucose, those numbers can help you determine the right amount of carbohydrate for you.

Regardless of how much carbohydrate you eat, the food choices you make are important.

- ▶ When choosing grains at breakfast, stick to high-fiber, whole-grain foods without added sugar, such as oatmeal, 100% whole-wheat toast, or quinoa.

- ▶ Fruit and low-fat dairy are also nutrient-dense carbohydrate foods that make great breakfast choices.

- ▶ If possible, include a source of protein such as eggs, nuts, nut butters, seeds, low-fat yogurt, low-fat milk, cottage cheese, or a lean breakfast meat. Adding protein may help you feel full for longer.

- ▶ Making a savory breakfast? Try adding some nutritious nonstarchy vegetables, such as tomatoes, peppers, mushrooms, and onions.

- ▶ Choose healthy fats, such as trans-fat-free margarine or peanut butter to spread on toast, nuts and seeds for mixing in oatmeal, or vegetable oil–based cooking spray when cooking your eggs.

Quick Grab-and-Go Options

Think there's no time to eat breakfast? Tired of eating the same old thing? Here are some meal ideas for you!

Egg Wrap or Breakfast Sandwich: Before you leave in the morning, crack an egg into a small microwaveable bowl or cup. Whisk it with 1 tablespoon of low-fat milk, black pepper, and a sprinkle of garlic powder. Heat the mixture in the microwave for 30 seconds to 1 minute, or until the egg is cooked through. Roll it up in a 6-inch whole-wheat tortilla along with a piece of reduced-fat cheese and pico de gallo. Or, put the cooked egg on a toasted whole-wheat English muffin to make a breakfast sandwich. Pack it in foil and take it with you in the car.

Oatmeal: It's a good whole-grain option. Keep some instant oatmeal packets at your house or at work. All it takes is adding some hot water and breakfast will be ready. You can also make a large batch of oatmeal on the weekend and reheat a cup in the microwave each morning.

Yogurt and Granola: On your way out the door, grab a cup of nonfat yogurt (regular or Greek) and a fruit and nut bar or granola bar.

Fruit and Cheese: Grab a small piece of fruit, such as an apple, banana, orange, pear, peach, or nectarine. Have it with a piece of string cheese.

Leftovers: Who says that you have to stick to conventional breakfast food? Did you make yourself a healthy dinner the night before? When cleaning up after dinner, pack leftovers in a container that you can grab on your way out the door the next morning.

Sample Breakfast Menus

You can add a cup of coffee or tea with a packet of artificial sweetener (if desired) to any of these menus without adding extra calories or carbohydrate.

Breakfasts with 30 Grams of Carbohydrate or Less

Cottage Cheese with Fruit and Nuts
   1/2 cup low-fat cottage cheese, *mixed with*
      1 peach, diced (or another small piece of fruit)
      1/4 cup unsalted dry-roasted almonds

Veggie Omelet and Whole-Wheat Toast
   Omelet *made with*
      1 whole egg
      2 egg whites
      1/2 cup sautéed green peppers and onions
      2 tablespoons reduced-fat cheddar cheese
   1 piece whole-wheat toast, *topped with*
      2 teaspoons trans-fat-free margarine

Toasted English Muffin and Strawberries

1/2 whole-wheat English muffin (toasted), *topped with*
>2 teaspoons trans-fat-free margarine

1 cup strawberries, *served on the side*

Banana and Peanut Butter

1 small (6-inch-long) banana, *served with*
>2 tablespoons peanut butter

Breakfasts with About 45 Grams of Carbohydrate

Oatmeal with Healthy Mix-Ins

3/4 cup cooked oatmeal (made with water, not milk), *mixed with*
>2 teaspoons brown sugar
>
>2 tablespoons dried cranberries or raisins
>
>1/4 teaspoon cinnamon
>
>1 tablespoon chopped pecans

Strawberry Banana Smoothie

Smoothie *made with*
>1/2 cup nonfat plain yogurt
>
>1/4 cup soy milk
>
>1/2 small banana
>
>1/2 cup frozen strawberries

10 walnut halves, *served on the side*

Cereal and Fruit

1 1/4 cup Cheerios (or a similar unsweetened whole-grain cereal), *served with*
>1/2 cup skim milk

1 small nectarine (or other piece of fruit), *served on the side or mixed in with cereal*

Breakfasts with About 60 Grams of Carbohydrate

Peanut Butter Toast with Grapefruit

1 slice whole-wheat toast, *topped with*

2 tablespoons peanut butter

1/2 grapefruit

1 cup skim milk

Waffles and Blueberry Yogurt Parfait

2 frozen whole-grain waffles (toasted), *topped with*

2 teaspoons trans-fat-free margarine

2 tablespoons sugar-free syrup

3/4 cup blueberries, *mixed with*

1/2 cup nonfat vanilla Greek yogurt

Quick Egg Wrap

1/3 cup egg substitute, *whisked together with*

2 tablespoons low-fat milk

scramble in a nonstick pan and wrap in

1 (10-inch) reduced-carb whole-wheat tortilla, *topped with*

1/4 cup diced tomato

2 slices avocado

1/4 cup black beans

1 cup strawberries, *served on the side*

Budget-Friendly Tip

If you are on a budget, then you're in luck! Many budget-friendly items at the grocery store are perfect breakfast options. Think peanut butter and toast, eggs, frozen and canned fruit, and oatmeal!

Snacks

When it is time for a snack, don't think salty chips, pretzels, or cookies. Snacking is really an opportunity to fit more nutritious foods into your day. When choosing snacks, focus on healthful foods, such as vegetables, fruits, whole grains, low-fat dairy, nuts, and seeds. These foods can give you an energy boost and will keep you feeling full until your next meal.

To Snack or Not to Snack?

Having diabetes does not mean you have to eat three meals and three snacks per day. Many adults can manage their diabetes without any snacks at all. Remember that eating when you are not hungry can lead you to take in extra calories and gain weight. But if your meals are spaced far apart or you tend to get hungry between meals, including a snack may be necessary. You may need to include snacks if you are very active and/or at risk for low blood glucose. Talk to your health-care provider about your schedule and preferences. They can help you decide if snacks should be included in your meal plan.

How much you eat for a snack will also depend on your plan. Often, sticking to around 15 grams of carbohydrate per snack is best. Still, many people with diabetes will eat an even lower-carbohydrate snack or may not need a snack at all.

How to Avoid Overeating at Snack Time

You'll also want to watch portions when snacking. It is easy to lose track of how much you eat, and you don't want to end up eating as many calories as you would have in a meal.

A lot of us tend to snack mindlessly in front of the television, computer, or while reading or driving. To avoid mindless eating, pre-portion snacks and eat from a smaller bowl, plastic bag, or plate. You can even use measuring spoons and measuring cups to be sure you don't over-serve yourself. Eating out of a family-size bag or bulk-size container can lead to overeating.

Snack Ideas

Check out some healthy snack ideas (with varying amounts of carbohydrate) below.

Snack	Carbohydrate (grams)
1 hardboiled egg	0
1/2 cup 2% low-fat cottage cheese + 3 tomato slices	6
2 cups light popcorn	10
1/2 toasted English muffin + 2 teaspoons trans-fat-free margarine	13
1 small to medium piece of fresh fruit	15
1/4 cup dry-roasted almonds + 1 tablespoon raisins, packed	15
1 cheese stick + 5 whole-wheat crackers	16
1 cup sliced cucumbers and celery + 1/4 cup hummus	16
1 small (4-ounce) apple + 1 tablespoon peanut butter	19
1 ounce pita chips + 2 tablespoons guacamole	20
1 cup raspberries + 1/4 cup light yogurt	20

Free Snacks

A "free food" is any food or drink choice that has fewer than 20 calories and has 5 grams of carbohydrate or less *per serving*. Free foods (and drinks) do not need to be counted in your diabetes meal plan as long as you have 3 servings or fewer spaced throughout the day.

If you are looking for something to tide you over between meals that won't affect your blood glucose or calorie intake, you can try one of the following free food* snacks:

➤ 3/4 cup light popcorn

➤ 1/2 cup sugar-free gelatin

➤ 6 grapes

➤ 5 baby carrots and celery sticks

➤ 1/4 cup blueberries

➤ 1/2 ounce fat-free cheese

➤ 8 goldfish crackers

➤ 4 black olives

➤ 1 frozen sugar-free cream pop

---

*adapted from *Choose Your Foods: Food Lists for Diabetes.* American Diabetes Association, 2014.

Pesto Hummus

Enjoy this hummus as a dip for snacking with nonstarchy vegetables, pita chips, or whole-wheat crackers.

Serves: 5 / Serving Size: 1/4 cup

1 (14.5-ounce) can garbanzo beans, drained and rinsed
2 tablespoons store-bought pesto
Juice of 1 small lemon (or 1/2 large lemon)
1 clove garlic, crushed
1/2 teaspoon freshly ground pepper

1. Add all ingredients to a food processor or blender. Blend until beans become a paste and ingredients are mixed well.

Nutrition Facts

Calories	100		**Potassium**	150	mg
Total Fat	3.0 g		**Total Carbohydrate**	14	g
Saturated Fat	0.4 g		Dietary Fiber	4	g
Trans Fat	0.0 g		Sugars	3	g
Cholesterol	0	mg	**Protein**	5	g
Sodium	155	mg	**Phosphorus**	80	mg

Exchanges/Food Choices

1 Starch, 1/2 Fat

Refreshing Cottage Cheese and Tomato

This is a simple and savory snack that you can enjoy when you need a quick pick-me-up.

Serves: 1 / Serving Size: About 1 cup

1/2 cup 2% cottage cheese
5 cherry tomatoes, quartered
3 large basil leaves, sliced into thin strips
Freshly ground pepper, to taste

1. Add cottage cheese to a small bowl and top with tomatoes and basil strips. Season with freshly ground pepper.

Nutrition Facts

Calories	110		Potassium	270	mg
Total Fat	3.0 g		Total Carbohydrate	7	g
Saturated Fat	1.1 g		Dietary Fiber	1	g
Trans Fat	0.0 g		Sugars	6	g
Cholesterol	10 mg		Protein	14	g
Sodium	375 mg		Phosphorus	205	mg

Exchanges/Food Choices

1 Vegetable, 2 Lean Protein

Easy, Heart-Healthy Snack Mix

Here's a heart-healthy snack mix that will keep you feeling full and energized until your next meal. Portion it out after you make it so it's easy to bring with you on-the-go.

Serves: 3 / **Serving Size:** 1/4 cup

1/4 cup dry-roasted, unsalted peanuts
1/4 cup dry-roasted, unsalted almonds
2 tablespoons golden raisins
3 dried apricots, chopped
3 snack-sized plastic baggies

1. In a small bowl, mix together the peanuts, almonds, raisins, and apricots.
2. Portion 1/4 cup of snack mix into each plastic baggie.

Nutrition Facts

Calories	175		Potassium	290	mg
Total Fat	12.0 g		**Total Carbohydrate**	14	g
Saturated Fat	1.3 g		Dietary Fiber	3	g
Trans Fat	0.0 g		Sugars	8	g
Cholesterol	0 mg		**Protein**	6	g
Sodium	0 mg		**Phosphorus**	110	mg

Exchanges/Food Choices

1 Fruit, 1 High-Fat Protein

Eating Out and Quick Meals

Don't have the time or energy to cook tonight? This is where managing diabetes can get tricky. With our busy schedules, eating out has become part of our daily lives. But restaurant and fast food is often loaded with calories, unhealthy fats, and sodium.

So what can you do? When you are eating at a restaurant or grabbing takeout, there are a lot of ways to make healthier choices. Remember to watch your portion sizes and try to choose options that best fit your meal plan.

Start with Portion Control

A major reason that restaurant foods are so high in calories, fat, and sodium is because the portions are so large. Keep portions in perspective by ordering the smallest sandwich. For example, go with the regular hamburger instead of the double bacon cheeseburger. Or order a 6-inch sub instead of the 12-inch sub. You could also order a lunch-size meal or a small plate.

Another idea is to save half of your meal for later. This is a good way to keep portions under control, and you'll also have a meal ready to go for lunch or dinner the next day.

To save calories and money, you could split your meal with a friend or family member. If you decide to spring for dessert, split one dessert with the entire table and savor a few bites to curb your sweet craving.

When you order takeout and bring it home, use the Diabetes Plate Method (see pages 31–32). Serve your food on a 9-inch plate and use this method to keep portions in perspective. You can also use the Diabetes Plate Method when you go to a restaurant that serves their food family style.

Order Wisely at Restaurants

Many restaurants have their menus and nutrition information online now. If possible, check the menu before you go out to eat so you can pick the best option ahead of time. This is especially helpful for checking the grams of carbohydrate in different meals. When you are choosing what to order, remember these tips:

> Choose a meal that includes nonstarchy vegetables! Ask for extra vegetables on your sandwich, order a side salad, or order a salad for your entrée.

> Choose meals where the meat or poultry is baked, broiled, roasted, or grilled. Avoid items that are fried.

> French fries, tater tots, and onion rings are fried and high in calories. Opt for more nutritious, lower-calorie side dishes, such as steamed vegetables, a garden salad with dressing on the side, baby carrots, apple slices, fruit salad, or low-fat yogurt.

> Ask for sauces and dressings on the side. Try dipping the tips of your fork prongs in the dressing or sauce and then get a bite of food. Or add one teaspoon of dressing at a time to your salad. Taste it before adding more so you avoid unnecessary calories. You'll be surprised how a little bit goes a long way.

> At sit-down restaurants, ask your server to have your meal prepared without using extra butter or salt. If an item is sautéed, ask if it can be sautéed lightly in olive oil rather than butter.

- Watch out for "freebies" on the table like bread or tortilla chips. These are high-carbohydrate foods and need to be counted in your meal plan if you decide to eat them. You can always ask your server to remove the temptation if you want to save your carbohydrate and calories for the main meal.

- Ask for low-calorie salad dressings, even if they are not on the menu. Vinegar with a dash of oil or a squeeze of lemon is also a better choice than high-fat dressings.

- Limit alcohol, especially high-calorie mixed drinks, which add calories but no nutrition to your meal.

A Quick Guide to Eating at Ethnic Restaurants

We have many restaurant options available to us now, including many ethnic restaurants. These restaurants do not always have nutrition information available for their menus, but you can still enjoy different cuisines. Here are some healthier options to look for at various types of restaurants:

At Mexican Restaurants:

- Ask the waiter to remove any fried tortilla chips from your table. That way, you won't be tempted to graze and can save your carbohydrate and calories for the main course.

- Some better-for-you options to look for include fajitas or tacos made with chicken, vegetables, or fish.

- When ordering, ask for soft tortillas rather than fried hard taco shells. Choose corn tortillas when possible, as they are usually made with whole grains.

- Get sour cream and cheese on the side and use these fixings sparingly.

- Try small sides of Mexican rice, black or pinto beans, and salsa. Note that refried beans are often made with lard, so ask the server how they are made before ordering.

At Chinese Restaurants:

▸ First of all, share! Dishes at these restaurants tend to be large. When dining in, ask your server for an empty plate that you can fill on your own, keeping portions and the Diabetes Plate Method in mind. If you order takeout, portion out your food on a plate at home instead of eating straight from the container.

▸ For a starter, try a cup of wonton, egg drop, or hot and sour soup. These are better choices than fried egg rolls, fried dumplings, or barbequed spare ribs.

▸ Steer clear of entrées that are fried, such as General Tso's chicken, fried rice, and dishes that are mainly noodles, like lo mein. Lightly stir-fried chicken, shrimp, tofu, or vegetable-based entrées are a much better option.

▸ Opt for steamed brown rice when available.

▸ Another issue with Chinese cuisine is the high-sodium sauces. Even low-sodium soy sauce is high in sodium, with over 500 mg in a tablespoon. Order steamed chicken, fish, and vegetable dishes with sauce on the side when possible. That way you control how much sauce is added.

▸ Ask for dishes to be prepared without extra salt, MSG, or large amounts of oil.

At Italian Restaurants:

▸ For an appetizer, try a broth-based soup, such as minestrone or Italian bean soup. Bruschetta or a house salad with dressing on the side are other good options.

▸ Opt for dishes with light marinara sauce or red clam sauce rather than creamy sauces, such as alfredo sauce.

▸ Look for an entrée that includes some nonstarchy vegetables.

▸ Main courses that are usually on the lighter side include grilled fish, chicken cacciatore, or shrimp scampi. Pasta primavera made with a red sauce or pasta with white or red clam sauce can also be good choices. These dishes are usually large, so try splitting entrées or see if a half order is available.

▶ Watch out for fried items and dishes that focus on just cheese, meat, and pasta, such as lasagna or chicken parmesan.

▶ Ask for whole-wheat pasta when available.

At Thai Restaurants:

▶ Try steamed mussels, kebobs, Thai shrimp soup, Thai salads, chicken with vegetables, garlic shrimp, or vegetables and tofu.

▶ The best options will include lots of nonstarchy vegetables.

▶ Ask for any rice on the side and opt for brown rice if available.

Cook When You Can

Keep in mind that going out for dinner used to be a special occasion. While fast food and takeout have made our lives easier, it can be challenging to find a healthy meal when eating out. But it is also hard to cook healthful meals at home if you don't have the ingredients on hand.

Plan ahead and stock your kitchen with the ingredients you need to make quick and healthy meals. On the weekend, look at your schedule for the next week. Pick out the days that you'll have time to cook dinner. When you can, plan to make extras so you can have the leftovers another night. On the weekend, for example, you can make a large batch of your favorite healthy chili or stew. Portion it out in single-serving containers and freeze it. Pull a container out at a later date when you need a quick meal.

Choose some quick and healthy recipes. A great place to start is the American Diabetes Association's website *Recipes for Healthy Living* at www.diabetes.org/recipes. If you're searching on the Internet or in a cookbook, look for recipes with the nutrition information included so you can easily see how to work a serving of the food into your meal plan. Make a list of what you need for these recipes and head to the store.

Fast Meals to Make at Home

Here are some basic, healthy meals that you can make in a matter of minutes—no recipe needed.

Rotisserie Chicken and Vegetables: Pick up a rotisserie chicken on your way home from work. Heat up a frozen vegetable medley (without added sauce) and serve the veggies and chicken with some quick-cooking brown rice or quinoa.

Egg and Veggie Wrap: Whisk together some eggs. Add a bit of milk, and scramble. Wrap the eggs up in a whole-wheat tortilla with sautéed onions, mushrooms, and a dash of hot sauce.

Light Tuna Salad: For a light dinner, drain canned tuna and mix it with some light mayonnaise and nonfat Greek yogurt to make tuna salad. Mix in some shredded carrots, diced celery, ground black pepper, and lemon juice to taste. Use large lettuce leaves as a wrap for your tuna salad, or enjoy it on whole-wheat crackers.

Super-Easy Slow-Cooker Meals: Slow cookers are another easy way to have a one-pot meal ready when you get home. Just toss the ingredients in before you leave in the morning and they'll cook slowly during the day while you are out.

Reading Nutrition Labels

Nutrition Facts labels are full of useful information. You can use them to check the carbohydrate grams and serving size of foods so you know how to count them in your meal plan. These labels also allow you to compare foods so you can make the best choices.

Recipes and Nutrition Facts

Look for recipe sources that provide you with the information you would find on packaged foods. One free online resource from the American Diabetes Association where you can find recipes and their nutrition information is *Recipes for Healthy Living* at www.diabetes.org/recipes.

How to Use the Nutrition Facts Label

1. First, look at the Serving Size found toward the top of the label. All of the amounts listed on the label are for that portion size. So, if you are going to have twice the serving size listed, you'll also be eating twice the calories, twice the carbohydrate grams, and so on.

2. Next, check the grams of Total Carbohydrate per serving. That is the number you will use if you are carbohydrate counting. Even if you don't count carbohydrate, this number can be helpful for gauging the amount of carbohydrate in different foods.

What About the Grams of Sugar?

The grams of total carbohydrate on the label include all types of carbohydrate: starch, sugar, and dietary fiber. You'll notice that the grams of sugar and dietary fiber are also listed out below the total carbohydrate. All types of carbohydrate affect blood glucose, so focus on the total amount listed rather than just grams of sugar. To learn more about the types of carbohydrate, go to Chapter 2 (page 5).

Other Important Parts of the Label

Calories

The number of calories per serving is important. Even when you choose healthy foods, calories count! If you are trying to maintain or lose weight, you should also keep a close eye on the calories per serving in the foods you buy. Compare similar foods and choose those with fewer calories.

Fat

Fat content should also be considered. In particular, you want to limit trans fat and watch saturated fat, especially if you need to lower your cholesterol level. Both of these types of fat are listed out separately under "Total Fat." Trans fat is the most harmful to us. To learn more about different types of fats, turn to Chapter 5 (page 25).

Sodium

This is another nutrient to watch. On average, Americans consume too much sodium—close to 3,400 mg per day. However, it is recommended that people with diabetes aim for less than 2,300 mg of sodium per day. (Some people with high blood pressure and other conditions may need less, but that is something to discuss with your health-care provider.) There are some foods you may not suspect that are high in sodium. Again, be sure to check labels so you can identify these hidden

Nutrition Facts

Serving Size 1 cup (53g/1.9 oz)
Servings Per Container About 8

Amount Per Serving

Calories 190	**Calories from Fat** 25

	% Daily Value**
Total Fat 3g*	**5%**
Saturated Fat 0g	**0%**
Trans Fat 0g	
Cholesterol 0mg	**0%**
Sodium 95mg	**4%**
Total Carbohydrate 36g	**12%**
Dietary Fiber 8g	**32%**
Sugars 13g	
Protein 9g	**14%**

Vitamin A 0%	•	Vitamin C 0%
Calcium 4%	•	Iron 10%

*Amount in Cereal. One half cup of fat free milk
contributes an additional 40 calories, 65mg sodium,
6g total carbohydrates (6g sugars), and 4g protein.
**Percent Daily Values are based on a 2,000 calorie
diet. Your Daily Values may be higher or lower
depending on your calorie needs.

	Calories:	2,000	2,500
Total Fat	Less than	65g	80g
Sat Fat	Less than	20g	25g
Cholesterol	Less than	300mg	300mg
Sodium	Less than	2,400mg	2,400mg
Total Carbohydrate		300g	375g
Dietary Fiber		25g	30g

Calories per gram:
Fat 9 • Carbohydrate 4 • Protein 4

sources and compare foods to make the best choice. To learn more about sodium, see Chapter 13 (page 69).

Ingredient List

The ingredient list is also a helpful tool. Ingredients are always listed in order by weight from greatest to least. You can check the ingredients to find products that contain all or mostly whole grains versus refined flours. You should also check the ingredient list if you have an allergy or to look for ingredients that you are trying to avoid, like hydrogenated oils.

More on Sugars and Fiber

Sugars

The grams of sugar listed on the label is not as useful as many would hope. This number includes both natural sugars and added sugars. So, if you only look at the amount of sugars on a label you might end up omitting certain healthy choices that contain natural sugars, such as fruits and dairy. You can tell if a food has added sugar by reading the ingredient list on the label. To read more about the different types of sugar, turn to Chapter 9 (page 47).

Fiber

Fiber is a part of plant foods that is not digested or, depending on the type of fiber, is only partially digested. Beans—such as kidney or pinto beans—fruits, vegetables, and grains are all good sources of fiber. Aim for about 25 grams of fiber per day for adult women and 38 grams per day for adult men.

What About Foods That Don't Have Labels?

Not all foods that you buy will have labels. In fact, many of the healthiest foods do not have labels, such as fresh fruits and vegetables. To count these types of foods in your meal plan, you'll want to have an idea of how large a serving is so you can estimate the carbohydrate count. Check out the quick guide below for serving sizes with about 15 grams of carbohydrate:

> ❯ 1/2 cup of frozen or canned fruit

> ❯ 1 small piece of fruit (about 4 ounces)

> ❯ 3/4–1 cup of berries

> ❯ 1 cup cubed melon

> ❯ 3 cups raw nonstarchy vegetables

> ❯ 1 1/2 cups cooked nonstarchy vegetables

> ❯ 1/2 cup potatoes or other starchy vegetable

For more serving sizes, check out Chapter 7 (page 37) on carbohydrate counting.

Beware of Net Carbs!

Many food manufacturers make claims about the carbohydrate content of food. There is no standard definition for terms like "net carbohydrate," "impact carbohydrate," or "digestible carbohydrate." To get these numbers, in most cases, manufacturers are subtracting fiber and sugar alcohols from the total carbohydrate. That makes foods appear lower in carbohydrate than they really are. In most cases, this calculation is not accurate and will likely underestimate how a food impacts blood glucose. Always look at the "Total Carbohydrate" on the Nutrition Facts label first. Checking your blood glucose can help you identify how a particular food affects you.

Weight Loss

Is Weight Loss Important for People with Diabetes?

If you have type 2 diabetes and are overweight, weight loss may help improve your blood glucose levels, especially if you have been diagnosed recently. Losing weight also helps reduce your risk of heart disease, lowers blood pressure, lowers triglyceride levels, and may improve other conditions, such as sleep apnea and even depression. If you are overweight, weight loss is important for your overall health whether you have diabetes or not.

Weight Loss for Those at Risk for Type 2 Diabetes

For those who are overweight and at high risk for type 2 diabetes, weight loss is very important. You are at an increased risk of developing type 2 diabetes if you:

> Are related to someone with type 2 diabetes

> Have high cholesterol

> Have high blood pressure

- Are overweight

- Are not physically active

- Have been diagnosed with prediabetes

- Are African American, Latino, Native American, a Pacific Islander, or Asian American

- Have cardiovascular disease

- Are aged 45 years or older

Many people think they have to lose a large amount of weight to prevent diabetes. But that is not true. An important research study called the Diabetes Prevention Program showed that losing about 7% of your body weight can decrease your risk of type 2 diabetes. If you weigh 180 pounds, that is about 13 pounds. If you weigh 250 pounds, that is about 18 pounds. It isn't easy, but losing a small amount of weight can give you a big health boost. Being able to delay or prevent diabetes is a huge health bonus.

If you have type 2 diabetes, your family is also at risk for the disease. Encouraging them to lose weight if they need to may help them to prevent or delay the onset of diabetes. Working as a family toward eating healthier foods, being more physically active, and losing weight together can improve everyone's health.

What Is Prediabetes?

Prediabetes is when your blood glucose is higher than normal but not high enough to be called diabetes.

Setting a Weight-Loss Goal

How much weight do you want to lose? If you ask many people this, they will tell you 30, 50, or even 100 pounds. While a larger goal may be your ideal, remember that losing 5–7% of your body weight (usually about 10–20 pounds) has huge health benefits. When setting goals, be realistic. Reducing your previous intake by just 100 calories a day leads to a 10-pound weight loss in a year's time.

It is easy to get frustrated when you don't see the scale move quickly enough. With reality television shows where participants lose 11 pounds in 1 week, you might be thinking, if they can do it, so can I. While most people *do* lose more weight the first 2 weeks of weight loss, most of that is fluid, and weight loss slows significantly after the initial weeks. Setting a goal of 1–2 pounds per week is a safe and realistic goal. For some people, 2 pounds a month may be more realistic. Try taking weight loss in 5-pound increments; start by setting a goal to lose 5 pounds.

Once you've achieved your first goal, set another. Remember, smaller weight losses can have a big health impact, so try to get out of the mindset that 10 pounds means nothing. It means a lot, especially if you continue to follow a healthier eating plan and can keep those pounds off.

As you are setting goals for what you eat, consider increasing your physical activity level. Exercise can help you maintain your muscle mass as you are losing weight and also helps burn calories. See Chapter 21 (page 117) for more information on exercise.

Where Do I Start?

Focus on making small changes. There are many ways to go about losing weight and only you can decide the best plan for you based on your lifestyle and food preferences. There is no one way to lose weight but avoiding fad diets is important; they are not long-term solutions. Making small, realistic changes can help you lose weight and keep it off.

Steps to Get Started

1. **Find out what you eat and how much you exercise.** That sounds silly, but most of us don't remember exactly what and how much we ate yesterday or even this morning. The best way to really know is to write down everything that you eat and drink for 3 days. This includes a nibble while fixing snacks for the kids after school or taking a taste while cooking. Try to pick 3 typical days—1 day on the weekend and 2 days during the week. Include any exercise or physical activity you do as well. As an example, include walks, dancing, playing basketball, raking leaves, and cleaning the kitchen on your list. It may also be helpful to make a note about the situation when you are eating or exercising. (What time was it? Were you alone or with someone else?) For some people, just writing

everything down gives them enough information to pinpoint the first small change to make.

2. **Take a critical look at what you wrote down and think about small changes you might be able to make.** Can you see where you might be able to cut back on your portions? For example, did you have more than 1 cup of pasta? Can you cut back to 2/3 cup? Did you have cookies for a snack? Is an apple an option? There are many ways to change your routine. Only you can decide which changes will be the best fit for you. In terms of exercise, are you exercising most days of the week? Are there times in your day you might be able to fit in a quick 10-minute walk?

3. **Take a look at when and why you are eating.** Are you a nighttime snacker? Are you hungry? Or are you eating because you feel bored, lonely, or frustrated? If you are eating when you aren't hungry, try to be more mindful. Take your time, enjoy your food, and be aware of how hungry you are. Keeping tabs on your hunger level can keep you from overeating. If you have diabetes, talk to your health-care team about how much flexibility you have with when and how much you eat.

Tips on Eating for Weight Loss

➤ Measure or portion out your food so you know exactly how much you are eating.

➤ For beverages, switch to low-calorie, sugar-free drinks, such as water, unsweetened tea, sugar-free lemonade, or diet soda. Avoid regular soda, sports drinks, sweet tea, and fruit punch.

➤ At mealtime, eat more nonstarchy vegetables. Fill half your plate with nonstarchy vegetables, such as salad, tomatoes, carrots, and broccoli.

➤ When cooking pasta, mix in some steamed fresh vegetables or cooked frozen veggies before adding your sauce. A cup of pasta mixed with veggies will have fewer calories than a cup of pasta alone.

➤ Start your meal with a side salad or a broth-based vegetable soup.

➤ Keep your portions very small when it comes to dessert.

➤ When eating out, be aware of portion sizes. Plan to take half your meal home for lunch the next day by requesting a take-home container before you start to eat. You could also split a meal with a friend.

➤ Switch to low-fat or nonfat milk and dairy products.

➤ For a snack, try unbuttered popcorn, reduced-fat string cheese, a hard-boiled egg, a piece of fresh fruit, a small handful of nuts, or veggies with bean dip.

➤ Keep fresh fruit on the counter so it is the first thing you see when you want a snack.

➤ If you drink alcohol, use low-calorie mixers, choose light beer over regular, and limit yourself to one drink per day for women and two per day for men. See Chapter 12 (page 65) for more on drinking alcohol if you have diabetes.

➤ If you tend to overeat on sweets, don't buy them or buy just one portion so you can have a treat without having more than you want in your cabinet. Plan to have dessert only when you are away from home. Split the dessert with a friend to keep yourself on track.

➤ If you are in a hurry, try a meal replacement bar or shake when you are on the go and don't have time for lunch.

Keeping Weight Off

For most people trying to lose weight, it is not their first attempt. If you find yourself trying to lose the same 10 pounds over and over again,

Time-Saving Tips

Try batch cooking a healthy recipe. Cook more than needed for one meal and put leftovers into single-serving containers. They'll be ready to go for lunch the next few days or can be frozen for a quick meal when you don't have time to cook.

When you return from the store with fresh veggies, clean and package them right away for snacks. They'll be ready to eat when you are hungry or can be easily packed for lunch.

you're not alone. There are two important things you can do to help keep the weight off:

1. Stick to your healthier lifestyle. You'll want to continue the changes you have made toward a healthier eating plan and exercise. Going back to old habits will make the pounds return. This is why making small changes is so important. You want to pick things you can keep doing without feeling deprived. If you get off track and notice the scale creeping up, don't panic or give up. Start to keep your food diary again and get back to your healthier lifestyle.

2. Be physically active. Exercise is even more important for keeping weight off than it is for losing the weight initially. Set a goal for at least 60 minutes of exercise at least 5 times a week.

If you are looking for a step-by-step guide to help you lose weight, we highly recommend *Diabetes Weight Loss Week by Week* by Jill Weisenberger, MS, RDN, CDE.

Dietary Supplements

Dietary supplements have become very popular and can be found just about everywhere. Supplements are not limited to products like vitamin and mineral pills. There are many "proprietary blends" of juices, extracts, and herbs that also qualify as dietary supplements.

People with diabetes are frequently targeted by supplement manufacturers who claim that certain products will improve blood glucose levels and overall health, and help with weight loss. There are no vitamins, minerals, or other supplements recommended for everyone with diabetes.

Are the Claims Too Good To Be True?

Keep in mind when you read a supplement label, if it sounds too good to be true, it probably is. Watch out for these signs that a product is over-promising its benefits:

> ➤ It promises improved blood glucose control.

> ➤ It promises quick results.

> ➤ It guarantees weight loss without changing what you eat.

- It claims to be a cure to stop aging.

- It uses testimonials to support the health claims.

- It recommends the supplement for everyone.

- The product materials tell you not to trust your health-care provider.

How Are Supplements Regulated in the U.S.?

The U.S. Food and Drug Administration (FDA) regulates dietary supplements, drugs, and food ingredients. Does it surprise you that supplements are under a different set of regulations than those for food or drugs? Supplements are not evaluated for safety or whether they actually work. The FDA does not review health claims made about supplements before the product is allowed on store shelves. In other words, no one is testing the product for safety or even to determine if it contains what the label claims! This also means that no one checks supplements to make sure they don't contain harmful or undeclared ingredients.

Under the Dietary Supplement Health and Education Act of 1994 (DSHEA):

- The dietary supplement manufacturer is responsible for ensuring that the product is safe before it is marketed.

- FDA is responsible for taking action against any unsafe dietary supplement product after it reaches the market.

How Can I Tell If Something Is a Supplement?

You can spot a supplement because it has a label that says "Supplement Facts" on the back. Food products contain a Nutrition Facts label on the packaging.

Supplements are also required to carry the disclaimer: "These statements have not been evaluated by the Food and Drug Administration. This product is not intended to diagnose, treat, cure, or prevent any disease."

If there are complaints, then fraudulent claims are investigated. From time to time, there are sweeps of websites and letters of warning are sent to companies when their products don't meet standards or they make unsubstantiated health claims.

Can Supplements Be Harmful?

While the thought of achieving better health with vitamins, herbs, and other supplements is tempting, the vast majority of supplements will not help manage diabetes. In some cases, they may be harmful because supplements are not a replacement for medical care. If you take supplements instead of getting medical treatment, blood glucose levels can remain high, increasing the risk of diabetes complications.

Talk with Your Health-Care Provider

If you are taking any supplements, be honest with your health-care provider. Some supplements can interfere with medications that you may be taking. If your health-care team knows everything you are taking, both over the counter and by prescription, together you can come up with the best treatment plan for you.

Common Supplements Promoted to Improve Diabetes

Omega-3 Supplements

Eating foods that contain omega-3 fatty acids is recommended by most health organizations, including the American Diabetes Association. Foods containing omega-3s include fish, walnuts, flax and flaxseed oil, and canola oil. Because eating foods high in omega-3s is thought to decrease inflammation and help prevent heart disease, supplement manufacturers are heavily marketing omega-3 and "fish oil" supplements.

What does the research say? A major study found that people with diabetes who took omega-3 supplements did not have a lower risk of heart events than those who did not take supplements. While research continues to examine omega-3 supplements, current recommendations are to include food sources of omega-3, but not pills, to reduce your risk of heart disease.

Antioxidants

Antioxidants are nutrients that help prevent damage to cells from pollutants like cigarette smoke. Antioxidants include fat-soluble vitamins A and E and water-soluble vitamin C. Fat-soluble vitamins are stored in your body. So if you take a large dose, they can stay in your body for a long time. Water-soluble vitamins, like vitamin C, are not stored, so if you get more than your body needs, your body gets rid of it in your urine.

Vitamin A was originally thought to prevent cancer but now there is concern that supplementation can result in increased risk of osteoporosis, hip fracture, and some cancers.

Vitamin E has been promoted to prevent heart disease and improve immune function. However, a large study that gave people vitamin E found that people did not have fewer heart attacks or fewer incidences of cancer than those who did not take it. A better choice may be to eat vitamin E–rich foods, such as vegetable oils, nuts, seeds, whole grains, green leafy vegetables, broccoli, kiwi, mangoes, tomatoes, and spinach.

Vitamin C is needed for your immune system to function and also for blood to clot. Vitamin-C deficiency in the U.S. is rare. Originally it was thought that vitamin-C supplements would help prevent cancer and heart disease. Studies have shown that vitamin C doesn't protect against cancer and, so far, it has not been shown to protect against heart disease. It is fairly easy to obtain vitamin C from food instead of turning to supplements. Food sources of vitamin C include citrus fruits, such as oranges, grapefruit, lemons, and limes, and other fruits and vegetables, such as peppers, kiwi, broccoli, strawberries, cantaloupe, baked potatoes, and tomatoes.

Antioxidants are found naturally in foods, especially plant foods. Plant foods contain natural chemicals called phytochemicals. Researchers think that all the phytochemicals in a single food work together to provide health benefits. That helps to explain why research shows that you get health benefits from eating whole foods—especially plant foods, such as fruits, vegetables, nuts, and whole grains—but you won't get those same benefits from a pill.

Vitamin D

Vitamin D has been promoted to both prevent and treat diabetes along with many other health conditions. Vitamin D is made in our skin when it is directly exposed to the sun (not through a window). With the increase in using sunscreen and for people with darker skin or people who live in areas with less sunlight, a vitamin-D deficiency is possible.

There isn't enough scientific evidence to support everyone taking vitamin-D supplements. However, your health-care provider can easily test for a vitamin-D deficiency with a blood test. If you have concerns about whether you are getting enough vitamin D, talk to your health-care provider.

Food sources of vitamin D include: fortified dairy products (in the U.S.), fatty fish (salmon, tuna, and mackerel), egg yolks, cheese, beef liver, mushrooms, and fortified cereal. Some other foods, such as orange juice, yogurt, soy milk, and margarine, may be fortified with vitamin D.

Chromium

Research has been divided on whether or not chromium helps manage blood glucose levels, or if it helps with blood cholesterol levels or weight loss. It seems to be most useful for people who are malnourished, not those with access to food. Because overall studies have not shown a benefit, it is not recommended that all people with diabetes take a chromium supplement.

Chromium-rich food sources include: broccoli, whole grains, grape juice, oranges, potatoes, garlic, basil, turkey, oysters, eggs, and lean beef.

Herbs and Spices

Herbs and spices have been used for centuries, not only for their aromatic and culinary properties, but also as medicines. Many herbs and spices are touted to improve blood glucose control and, in some cases, cure diabetes.

One of the most common spices said to affect diabetes is cinnamon. Some research studies have looked at cinnamon and its effect on blood glucose, blood pressure, and cholesterol levels. However, results from these studies have been conflicting and of poor quality. To date, there is not enough evidence from research to claim that including large doses of cinnamon in your daily diet will help regulate blood glucose in people with diabetes. If you enjoy the taste of cinnamon, by all means, sprinkle it on your oatmeal, fruit, or toast.

Fresh herbs and roots, such as garlic, basil, cilantro, parsley, ginger, and mint, are a wonderful way to flavor food without added salt and fat. Like all plant foods, they contain phytochemicals that are good for us. Use them when you cook or try making ginger or mint tea for a calorie-free drink. Unfortunately, eating them by the spoonful is not going to improve your diabetes management, but they can do wonders for your taste buds!

For more information, visit the National Institutes of Health's Office of Dietary Supplements website at ods.od.nih.gov.

Exercise

Why Is Exercise Important?

Good nutrition and exercise go hand-in-hand when it comes to controlling diabetes. When you combine healthy eating, meal planning, and exercise, it can have a big impact on your weight, diabetes management, and overall health.

Regular exercise can:

> Lower your blood pressure and cholesterol levels

> Lower your risk for heart disease and stroke

> Burn calories to help you lose or maintain weight

> Make insulin work better

> Increase your energy for daily activities

> Help you sleep better

> Relieve stress

> Strengthen your heart

> Improve your blood circulation

- Strengthen your muscles and bones
- Keep your joints flexible
- Improve your balance to prevent falls
- Reduce symptoms of depression
- Improve your quality of life

For people with diabetes, the recommended goal is to get at least 30 minutes of moderate-intensity aerobic exercise, 5 days per week (or 150 minutes total). Try not to take more than 2 days in a row off from doing aerobic exercise. You'll also want to do some type of strength training 2 or more days per week.

What Counts as "Moderate-Intensity" Aerobic Activity?

Moderate intensity means that you are working hard enough that you can talk, but not sing, during the activity. Vigorous intensity means you cannot say more than a few words without pausing for a breath during the activity.

Get Started Safely and Slowly!

Exercise, or physical activity, includes anything that gets you moving, such as walking, playing tennis, or working in the yard. If you are not very active now, it's important to start slowly. Try starting with 5–10 minutes a day of activity and increase your activity sessions by a few minutes each week. Over time, you'll find that you are able to be active for longer and that you can increase your intensity. It is also important to choose activities that you enjoy. When you do, you'll be more likely to keep up with your routine.

Depending on your age and type of diabetes, or if you have complications such as heart disease or neuropathy, your health-care provider may tell you to avoid certain activities. In some cases, your health-care provider may need to do some tests as well.

Exercise and Hypoglycemia

People with type 1 diabetes are at the highest risk for hypoglycemia during and for several hours after exercise. If you have type 2 diabetes and are on insulin or an insulin secretagogue (a pill that makes your body release insulin), exercise can increase your risk for hypoglycemia as well. If you fall into these categories, don't be discouraged—the many benefits of exercise outweigh the risks. You'll just need to take a few precautions:

> ➤ Talk to your health-care provider about how to balance your insulin or medicine with physical activity. This may mean lowering your insulin dose or eating some extra carbohydrate before exercising to keep your blood glucose in a safe range.
> ➤ Learn how different types of activity affect you. Frequently check your blood glucose before, during, and after exercise sessions.
> ➤ If your blood glucose is below 100 mg/dl before exercising, have a snack with carbohydrate and do not exercise until your blood glucose is in the desired range.
> ➤ Always carry a source of carbohydrate with you that you can eat or drink quickly. Some good ideas are glucose tablets, glucose gel, or regular Gatorade.
> ➤ Always wear a diabetes ID when exercising.

Important Types of Activity

Aerobic exercise is anything that gets your heart pumping, like brisk walking, biking, dancing, swimming, or playing a sport. If you find it hard to fit in 30 minutes straight of aerobic activity, you can split it up into spurts of 10 minutes or more. For example, do 10 minutes of brisk walking in the morning before work, during your lunch break, and after dinner. Or try 15 minutes during the day and then 15 minutes after work. Make it work with your schedule!

Strength training helps you build strong muscles and bones. Some strength training activities include lifting weights, using resistance bands, calisthenics like pushups and sit-ups, or Pilates.

You should also take any opportunity to add more activity into your day. Take the stairs instead of the elevator. Walk in place during commercials when you watch TV. Or get up once an hour at work and take a quick lap around the office. The possibilities are endless.

Does Walking Count?

Yes! For most people, walking is a great way to start getting more active. Here are some advantages of walking for exercise:

> ➤ It doesn't require a gym membership or fancy equipment.
> ➤ It's an easy place to start since most of us do it every day—there's no learning curve!
> ➤ It has been shown to improve blood pressure, cholesterol, stress, and depression.
> ➤ It can help with weight management.
> ➤ It is a form of exercise that is easy to keep up—there are lots of places you can do it!

Wearing a pedometer is a good way to track how much you move during the day. A pedometer is an inexpensive tool that counts your steps when you clip it to your belt or waistband. You can buy one at most athletic stores or you can order one online. At the end of each day, check your pedometer and record your steps for the day.

Keeping a record of your steps can help you gauge how much activity you are getting or how far you are walking each day. It also gives you a starting point to help you set goals. Let's say you are getting around 2,000 steps per day. You can gradually increase your steps or the minutes you walk each day from there. You might set a goal to increase your average steps by 500 each week until you are getting 10,000 steps per day.

Busting Barriers

Keeping up an exercise routine is not always easy, and life can often get in the way. But it is important for your health to stay motivated and keep it up. Here are some solutions to common barriers to exercise.

Barrier #1: "30 minutes is too much. I don't have that kind of time." **Solution:** Do as much as you can. Every step counts! Split it up into three 10-minute bouts of exercise and do them throughout the day. You'll still see the same benefits.

Barrier #2: "I get bored when I exercise."
Solution: Choose activities that you enjoy. You might not like to jog or bike, but perhaps you like to play a team sport, or perhaps you love gardening. You can also try working out with music, in a class setting, or with a loved one to make it more enjoyable. Varying the activities you do can also help.

Barrier #3: "I'm too tired after work to exercise."
Solution: Find a time when your energy is highest and plan to do something active then. Or try breaking the exercise up into multiple small sessions of at least 10 minutes each. You don't have to go for a 10-mile run. A simple brisk walk counts as aerobic exercise and can be a great stress-reliever! Remember that increasing your activity level will also increase your energy over time.

Barrier #4: "I can't afford to join a fitness center or buy equipment."
Solution: Do something that doesn't require fancy equipment or a gym. Some good ideas are walking, dancing, calisthenics, or using water bottles for weights. Exercise bands are another inexpensive option. You can also look for a TV exercise program or find free exercise videos on the Internet or at the public library to do at home.

Barrier #5: "I'm afraid I'll get low blood glucose."
Solution: People who use insulin and those who take certain diabetes pills need to be the most concerned about low blood glucose from exercise. You should always be prepared. Make sure you have some glucose tabs, or another fast-acting carbohydrate to treat a low if one should occur. If you are worried, check your blood glucose to see how exercise affects you.

Barrier #6: "I don't have the motivation to exercise."
Solution: Planning out when you will exercise and what activity to do ahead of time is important. Invite a family member or join a group to exercise with on a regular basis. Involving others and having a routine can help keep you motivated and accountable. Setting goals and writing them down can also help.

Barrier #7: "I haven't exercised in years. I don't know where to start."
Solution: If you haven't exercised recently, don't let that stop you.
Just start slowly. Try walking for 5–10 minutes a day to start. You can increase the amount you walk by a few minutes each week. Try using a pedometer to track your progress. If you feel unsure about your health, check with your health-care provider before making big changes in your exercise plan.

Barrier #8: "Even walking is not an option for me."
Solution: There are still many exercise options, such as chair exercises or certain activities in the swimming pool, for people who need to avoid walking. Talk to your health-care provider about what type of exercises will be best for you.

Key Takeaways

1. Start slowly if you haven't been active for a while. If you are unsure about your health, talk to your health-care provider about what is safe for you.
2. People with diabetes should aim for at least 150 minutes of moderate-intensity aerobic exercise per week and include at least 2 strength training sessions per week.
3. Take any opportunity to add more activity into your day, from taking the stairs to parking at the back of the lot.

We hope you have enjoyed the book and that it has provided practical guidance on what to eat with diabetes. The American Diabetes Association has endless resources on all aspects of managing diabetes. On the following page, we've listed a few of our favorites.

—Stephanie and Cassie

Resources

American Diabetes Association
  1701 North Beauregard Street
  Alexandria, VA 22311
  1-800-DIABETES
  703-549-1500
  www.diabetes.org
  www.shopdiabetes.org

Internet Resources

Recipes for Healthy Living
  www.diabetes.org/recipes

Print Resources

American Diabetes Association: *Count Your Carbs: Getting Started*. Alexandria, VA, American Diabetes Association, 2014

American Diabetes Association: *Match Your Insulin to Your Carbs*. Alexandria, VA, American Diabetes Association, 2014

Hayes C: *The "I Hate to Exercise" Book for People with Diabetes*. 3rd ed. Alexandria, VA, American Diabetes Association, 2013

Newgent J: *The All-Natural Diabetes Cookbook*. Alexandria, VA, American Diabetes Association, 2007

Riolo A: *The Mediterranean Diabetes Cookbook*. Alexandria, VA, American Diabetes Association, 2010

Rondinelli-Hamilton L, Bucko Lamplough J: *Healthy Calendar Diabetic Cooking*. 2nd ed. Alexandria, VA, American Diabetes Association, 2012

Weisenberger J: *Diabetes Weight Loss Week by Week*. Alexandria, VA, American Diabetes Association, 2012